F

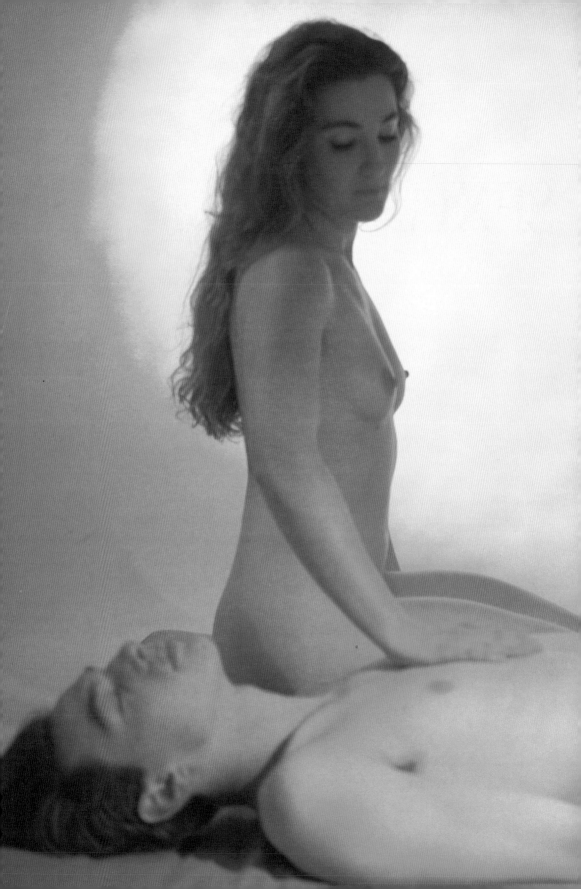

The Tao of
SEXUAL MASSAGE

Stephen Russell
and Jürgen Kolb

A Fireside Book
Published by Simon & Schuster Inc.

New York   London   Toronto   Sydney   Tokyo   Singapore

A GAIA ORIGINAL

Conceived by   *Joss Pearson*

Editorial   *Eleanor Lines*

Design   *Dave Thorp*

Photography   *John Hÿtch*

Illustration   *Gillian Hunt*

Direction   *Joss Pearson*

Patrick Nugent

FIRESIDE
Simon & Schuster Building
Rockefeller Center
1230 Avenue of the Americas
New York, New York 10020

Reproduction by Fotographics Ltd., Hong Kong, and Technographic Design and Print Ltd., Suffolk
Printed and bound by Mateu Cromo, Madrid, Spain

10 9 8 7 6 5

Library of Congress Cataloging-in-publication Data
Russell, Stephen, 1954-
The Tao of sensual massage/Stephen Russell with Jürgen Kolb
p. cm.
"A Fireside book"
Includes bibliographical references and index
ISBN 0-671-78089-1
1. Massage   I. Kolb, Jürgen.   II. Title
RA780.5.R875 1992
615.8'22--dc20   *91-44833 CIP*

How to use this book

The Tao of Sexual Massage introduces you to the art of using simple massage techniques to stimulate the fundamental energy in your body - your sexual energy. It is for everyone who is interested in improving the quality of their sexual experience.

Part One describes Taoist philosophy and the early Chinese medical tradition. The first chapter introduces the basic theory and describes how this is used in Taoist sexual practice. Chapter Two explains why we need sexual massage, and how it helps. Chapters Three and Four prepare you mentally and physically for the sequence that follows.

Part Two demonstrates the sequence of the massage, which is presented in two sections: first, the Back Sequence in Chapter Five, and second, the Front Sequence in Chapter Six.

If you want, begin straightaway by learning the Postural and Navel Breathing Meditations on pages 66-7. Then learn the basic massage techniques on pages 77-82. Turn to page 94 to begin the sequence.

Caution

In general this massage should not be performed by people with any condition that is currently being treated or needs treatment by a medically qualified doctor. Do not give or receive a massage if you are suffering from any contagious or infectious diseases. If you are pregnant, consult your physician before giving or receiving any of the techniques described in this book. Since this massage is normally performed on the floor, people with back complaints or injuries should not give this massage.

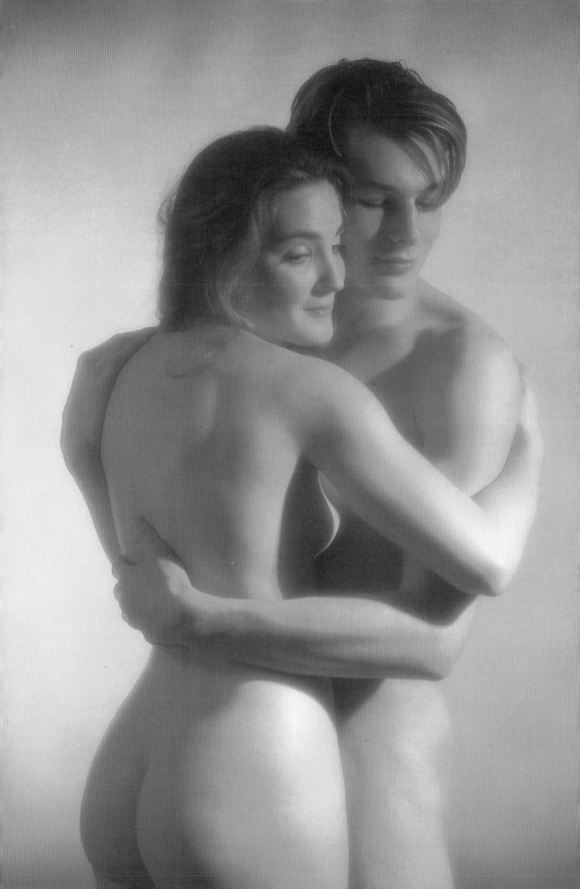

CONTENTS

Foreword   8

Introduction   10

Part One

Chapter One

Energy in Your Body   20

Chapter Two

Your Sexuality   44

Chapter Three

Preparing Yourself   60

Chapter Four

Before You Begin   68

Part Two

Chapter Five

Manual of Techniques: Back Sequence   92

Chapter Six

Manual of Techniques: Front Sequence   130

Treating Common Ailments   186

Bibliography, Acknowledgements, and Resources   188

Index   189

FOREWORD

I am very pleased to be associated with this book on Taoist massage.
Stephen Russell and I have worked together since 1983 and
throughout this time we have successfully combined Stephen's
teaching on Taoist medicine and massage with my work as an
obstetrician, managing the prenatal and postnatal care of mothers,
fathers, and babies. Stephen's teaching style, which is evident in this
book, is clear, exhilarating, and inspiring.

Massage is one of the most powerful forms of communication
between adults and also between parents and their newborn babies

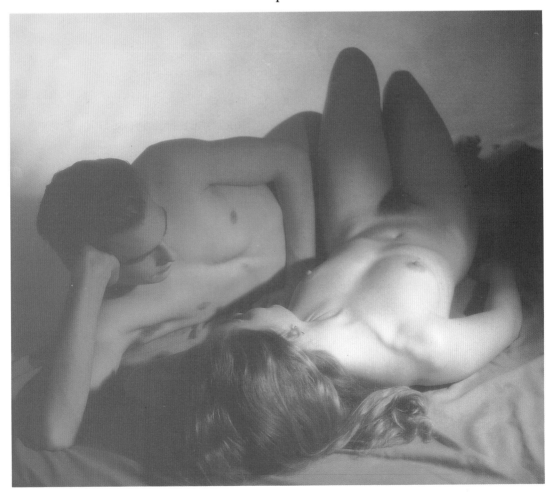

during the period from conception to the months after birth. Touch provides an additional dimension to the vision of the developing personality in the new born and helps us to experience the bond with our babies.

As adults, many men and women find it difficult to receive touch with warmth, grace, and openness. But this deep communication within a sexual relationship can be one of the peak experiences of life. Taoist philosophy can embrace the necessity for contact and intimacy throughout the life cycle - from the tactile needs of a new baby to the more intimate touch of adults.

This book teaches the principles of Taoist philosophy and energy flow in a simple, well illustrated way that is easy to understand. It offers readers a gentle guide into the exploration of their own energy field as well as that of their partners. Taoist massage is primarily designed to relax and encourage the energy flow of the participants, making the ability to give and to enjoy the act of making love infinitely easier and more satisfying.

This book is also about giving and receiving; it is about trusting and being trusted; it is about showing and accepting dependence and independence. It is a practical book that encourages and allows the uninitiated to learn quickly and effectively. Every couple will benefit deeply from discovering the magic of the Taoist inspired flow of energy.

Yehudi Gordon MD FRCOG

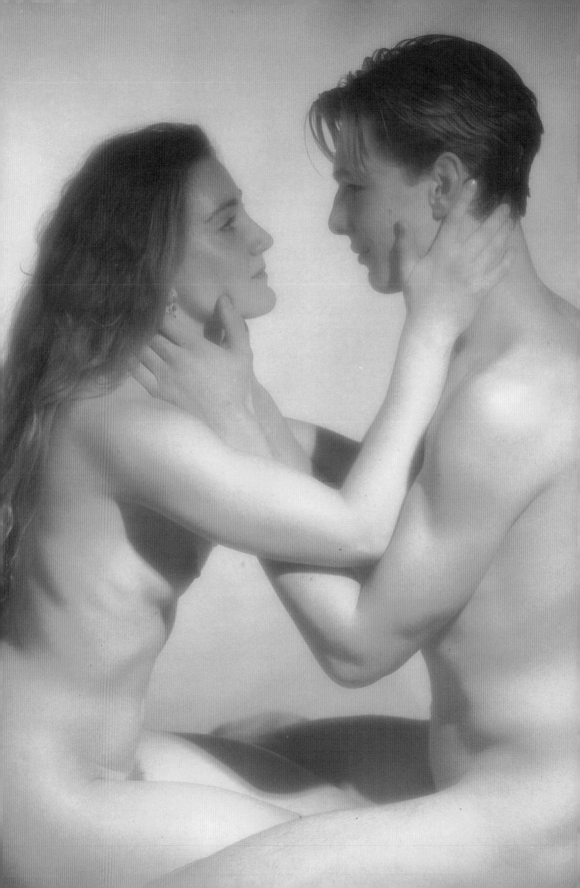

INTRODUCTION

In our primitive state, the sexual urge is as natural as the urge to eat food and breathe air. Primitive cultures acknowledge and even honour it in daily life as an expression of the basic life force. Where a less primitive culture has developed, our way of dealing with the sexual urge has been to suppress it, and to rechannel it into other areas of our lives. But sexual energy is the fundamental energy of the body. It provides the basis for all other types of energy, from the physical energy to survive, to the spiritual energy we need to continue our development. Taoist sexual massage clears the way for our sexual energy to circulate freely in the body and promote good health, peace of mind, and a fulfilling sexual experience. The massage system described in this book is the most comprehensive Taoist tool for achieving a healthy integration of sex into daily life.

Giving or receiving a sexual massage unifies the mind and body, and enables you to take this feeling into making love. It alters your level of awareness, heightening your feelings so that, with practice, the massage enables you to control and extend your enjoyment and the moments of ecstasy. Once you have gained this control, you can learn to take your consciousness beyond your physical form as you make love, and to celebrate the union with the Spirit that is present in us all. When this happens, you are transforming your sexual energy and using it in a spiritual way. This transformation of sexual energy into spiritual energy is the ultimate aim of Taoist sexual practice. *The Tao of Sexual Massage* enables the reader to work with this fundamental sexual energy, strengthening it, improving its circulation around the body, and transmuting it into spiritual energy.

Sex in relationships

This book is based on the authors' work as healing practitioners. As Freud and Reich found before us, so we have found that sexual disharmony, whether or not the root cause, is nonetheless fundamental to most forms of mental and physical disorder, both in the case of the individual and in society at large.

In our extensive work with couples we have discovered that once the initial ardour has worn off, relationships soon become sexually stagnant. We have taught this massage system to many couples and individuals, and have witnessed remarkable results with it. For couples whose sexual communication has become repetitive or even non-existent, the massage provides a new avenue through which to explore and revitalize sex, and increase the sex drive to a comfortable level. Moreover, it will sensitize you as a lover and enable you to draw more pleasure from the sexual experience. For single people, whether hetero- or homosexual, male or female, young or old, this book presents a different approach to sexual experience, which does not necessitate intercourse. This change in approach is important. The book represents a safe and practical way to pass on the essence of the Taoist healing wisdom.

What is the Tao?

Contemporary Taoist teachings encapsulate all the wisdom of the ancient sages, based on information passed down to the Chinese from a legendary culture, known by some as the Sons of Reflected Light, about 14,000 years ago. Taoist teachings contain a high degree of mystification in their explanations. The most famous of all Taoist aphorisms is "the Tao which can be explained is no longer the Tao". It is our intention, while describing the sexual massage system and philosophy in this book, to help to demystify the meaning of the Tao.

The word Tao, translated from Chinese, simply means "The Way". In the context of Taoist cosmology however, it has a far deeper meaning. Tao means both existence and the state of non-existence from which it springs. Tao refers to the Great Way of the Universe. Underlying this is the concept of the Tao as the consciousness at the heart of manifest and nonmanifest existence. It is this same consciousness that leads the grass to grow, planets to turn, and stars to shine. The Tao is also the consciousness at the depth of your very being. Infinitely creative - from a sperm to a universe, from a passing thought to an eon of history - it is the Tao

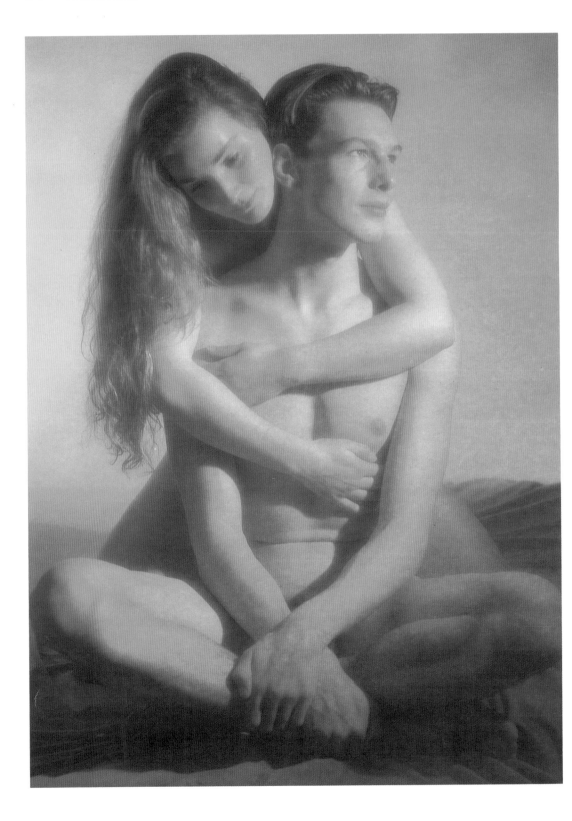

that has created them all. It is also the Tao that has guided us to write this book, and you to read it.

You cannot see or feel the Tao, it is everywhere and nowhere at the same time. Although you are indistinguishable from it, you will never be able to know or understand such an all-encompassing concept of existence. Its totality just cannot be known. But if you can still your mind and sink your awareness deep enough, to a point of magnificent inner silence, you will be it.

Oneness with the Tao

Through the millennia, the aim of Taoist spiritual masters and sages has been to achieve this oneness with the Tao. However, oneness is not something that can be fully grasped by the intellect. It depends on intellect giving way to feeling, on your ability to focus on the sensations in your body - of warmth, of safety, of happiness - rather than on your thoughts. In periods of intense activity, when your mind is free from noise and interference, when your thoughts are focused only on what you are doing, and your mental and physical activities are working together, you can be at peace with yourself and the rest of the world. In this state you can think, move, and feel as a unified being. Many of the Taoist techniques such as meditation, martial arts, long-distance running, and yoga exercises were specifically designed as tools for achieving this.

The sexual union of love-making heightens your feelings and reduces the work of your intellect. Ultimately, in the moments of orgasm, you can experience oneness with the Tao. It is a fleeting glimpse of the Absolute. In such a moment you are enlightened.

Freedom and the Tao

By nature, Taoism is gentle, responsive, and without rules and regulations. Taoist philosophy has always claimed that change is fundamental to existence. The natural dynamic in life provides a constant ebb and flow in events and in our lives. No sooner has a situation arisen than it has gone. No set of rules, however elaborate, can guide us through all the eventualities of our lives. Taoism bestows the freedom from restrictive conventionality, and gives licence to respond to life in whatever way is necessary. Emphasis is placed on the performance of positive health-enhancing techniques and not on a long list of prohibitions. Taoism is simply an attitude of being natural - like a child - playing in life, whether working or resting.

Synthesis of east and west

Our background is in healing, as practitioners of meditational, martial, and healing arts, as well as in the western psycho-therapeutic approach and in hypno-therapeutic work. We have witnessed a natural synthesis of these eastern and western systems in our practices. Our discoveries, culled from many hours of clinical practice, are passed on in this book.

The translation of Taoist names

During the course of this book you will come across, or maybe stumble over, many Taoist names for certain areas of the body and the psyche. It is common practice among teachers of the Tao to employ several names for one particular part of the psycho-physical map. For example, the area toward the back of the head, directly on top of the upper brainstem, is variously called: The Upper Tan T'ien, The Ni Wan Palace (Nirvana Palace), The Terrace of the Ancestors, The Terrace of the Living, The Home of the Great Void, The Cave of the Original Spirit, and many titles far more imaginative. The reason for this interchanging of names is probably related to differences in translation from the original Chinese. Some teachers also believe that different names were introduced deliberately, to loosen up the student's mind. For the sake of clarity in the context of this book, we have endeavoured wherever possible to use just one name for each area.

We would like you to come to this book with a relaxed attitude of light concentration. It is as much for your increased sexual enjoyment as for your progress along a spiritual path. If you want, skip over the philosophical explanation in Chapters One and Two, and try the massage straightaway. Do not feel daunted by the sequence of the massage presented in Part Two of this book. If you decide to try one or two isolated techniques at first you can be sure that the results are bound to please.

Stephen Russell

Jürgen Kolb

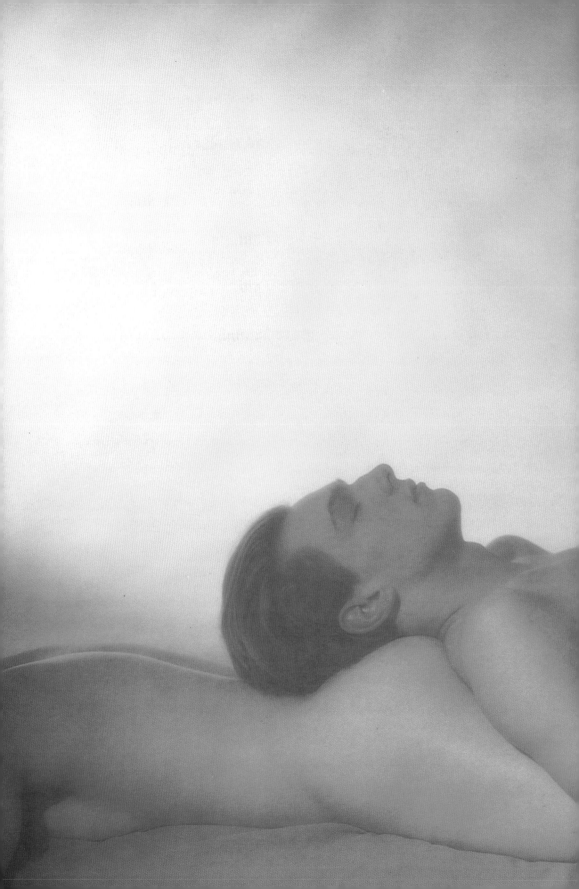

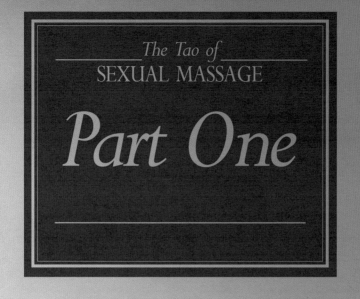

The Tao of
SEXUAL MASSAGE

Part One

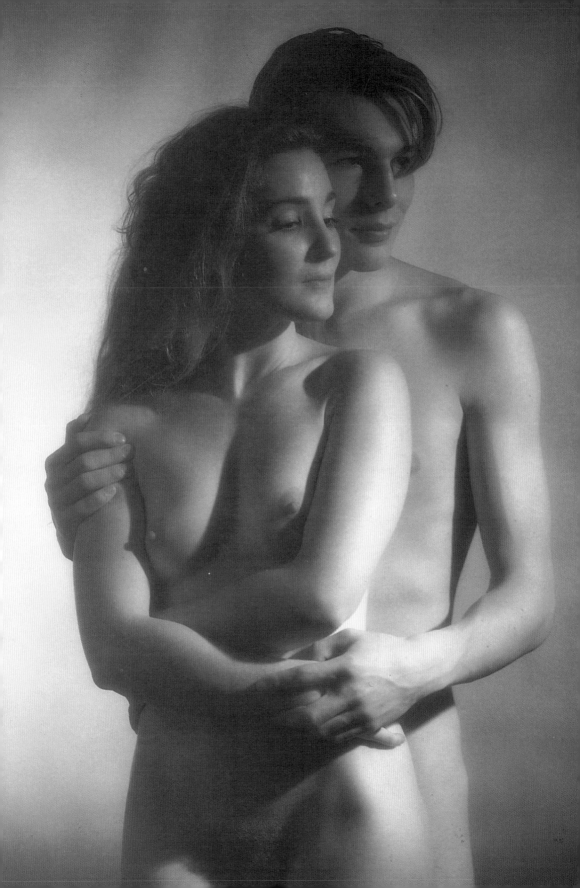

Chapter One

ENERGY IN YOUR BODY

THE Taoist interpretation of body energy is explained simply and clearly in this chapter. It will change your view of how your body functions. Everything that we experience is created from Yin and Yang forces (see pp. 22-3), and the more refined Five Element theory (see pp. 24-5) explains the interconnectedness of all phenomena. The energy that flows through our bodies under the influence of Yin and Yang and the Five Elements, and which connects us with the universe, is described on pages 26-9.

The theory behind Taoist sexual massage is based on the role of sexual energy in the body (see pp. 26-33). As sexual energy circulates around the body (see p. 34), it is transformed into other types of energy, including spiritual energy. The massage sequence in Part Two helps this circulation and transformation of the energy. Ultimately, you can control this energy, not only during the massage, but while making love, turning this union into a deeply spiritual experience (see pp. 35-7).

Chapter One ends by describing some advanced Taoist practices for using your powerful spiritual energy as a healing force (see pp. 38-40), and techniques for enhancing its availability.

The Yin and the Yang

According to Taoist cosmological belief, all existence, whether manifest or nonmanifest, evolves from the eternal struggle of two opposing forces: the Yin - female, dark, inward-moving, and receptive; and the Yang - male, bright, outward-moving, and active force.

One of the most fundamental philosophical achievements of the ancient Taoist sages was the realization that existence cannot be observed beyond the duality of these two opposing cosmic powers. The forces of Yin and Yang are seen to permeate all existence. Existence, both manifest and nonmanifest, is made possible by the interplay of these two polar forces, travelling through all dimensions in opposite directions. It is the friction between these two energies, as they constantly pass through each other, that generates our manifest existence, the material world and everything that we experience, or what Taoists sometimes call the "Ten Thousand Things" (see p. 24).

Yet the velocity with which the forces of Yin and Yang permeate each other, as they pass in opposing directions, is not consistent. There is a tidal motion: an ebb and flow. It is in this cross current that you are born and live, subject to the ever changing powers that surround you.

The forces of Yin and Yang operate within your physical form as well as around it. It is the earth-bound, inward-moving, imploding Yin energies within you that give substance to your body. It is the space-bound, outward-moving, exploding Yang energies within you that give motivation to your body. Substance without motivation is inert mass, and motivation without substance goes nowhere.

Yin and Yang, like light and shadow, are mutually interdependent. Any cessation in the ebb and flow between

YIN
Night
Form
Wet
Cold

The relationship between Yin and Yan

them leads to a Yin illness, when the body fluids coagulate, or a predominantly Yang illness, in which the body fluids overheat and dry up. When the ebb and flow stops for long enough, you no longer conduct the two energies, and you die.

Any rigidity or stiffening in your physical body or mental attitude blocks the flow of Yin and Yang energy (see Chapter Two) and will in time speed the ageing and death processes.

**YIN
WITHIN
YANG**

**YANG
WITHIN
YIN**

YANG
Daylight
Force
Dry
Hot

Yin and Yang
Yin is neither good nor bad.
Yang is neither good nor bad.
They are simply two opposing and
complementary forces of existence.
The interplay between them causes
new growth. The harmony between
them causes great peace.

The Five Elements, and the creation of the Ten Thousand Things

The Tao is the indivisible. For creation to occur, the indivisible must divide. The One - the Tao - becomes Two, the Yin and Yang (see p. 22). The interplay of Yin and Yang, also known as "The World of Opposites", creates a force composed of five mutually supporting, controlling, and inter-checking elements. These are Water, Wood, Fire, Earth, and Metal (see illustration, facing page). The movement of this combined force produces the manifest world of phenomena, or what Taoists call the "Ten Thousand Things". Every phenomenon of existence encapsulates this creative process.

In human affairs, women and men are personifications of the basic Yin and Yang dichotomy. The actions of both sexes are coloured by the interplay of five basic emotions, each of which corresponds to one of the Five Elements. These emotions are: fear (Water), anger (Wood), excitement (Fire), sadness (Earth), and longing, or grief (Metal). The combined result of this is the life and world you live in.

Normally, in a healthy, balanced individual, these five emotions rise and fall continuously, in various combinations, producing a richness and variation of emotional experience. When two such balanced and healthy people interact in a relationship together this interplay of the five emotions becomes synergistic; their relationship is happy and creative. In most people, however, one of the emotions will dominate. This both arises out of and causes a block in the body's energy. Such a block diminishes the ability for friction-free and easy socialization. Needless to say, if two people

Five Element associations
Each element (top) is most closely linked with a particular organ. Th... is paired with an associated organ. Together, these organs and the element control a person's physical and emotional aspects as well as being responsible for a part of the energy production in the body.

Generating and controlling sequences
The elements are linked to each other in two distinct ways. The arrows around the outside show a progression from one element and pair of organs to another. This reflects the direction of energy flow through the organs. The arrows within the circle demonstrate the control exerted by each element an... pair of organs over another.

with such energy blocks try to make a partnership, the relationship will not be an easy one.

The sexual massage that follows in Part Two works on the basic energy field and, by clearing it, reconstitutes the balance between the five emotions and elements. This in turn balances the interplay of man and woman, Yin and Yang.

The Five Elements

There is a large body of knowledge within Taoist medicine and philosophy concerning the interactions of the Five Elements. Countless implications for life, health, and the functioning of the world have been studied and recorded.

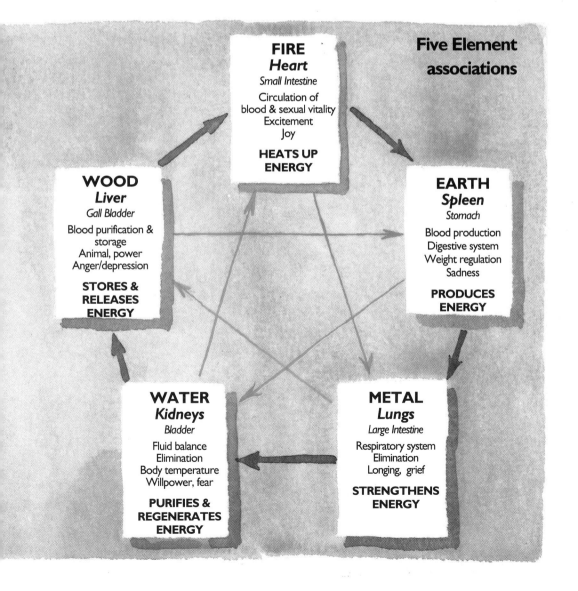

Five Element associations

FIRE
Heart
Small Intestine
Circulation of blood & sexual vitality
Excitement
Joy

HEATS UP ENERGY

WOOD
Liver
Gall Bladder
Blood purification & storage
Animal, power
Anger/depression

STORES & RELEASES ENERGY

EARTH
Spleen
Stomach
Blood production
Digestive system
Weight regulation
Sadness

PRODUCES ENERGY

WATER
Kidneys
Bladder
Fluid balance
Elimination
Body temperature
Willpower, fear

PURIFIES & REGENERATES ENERGY

METAL
Lungs
Large Intestine
Respiratory system
Elimination
Longing, grief

STRENGTHENS ENERGY

The human energy field

To understand the full potential of sexual massage, it helps to know something about the Taoist notion of the energy field, which permeates human beings and all existence. According to Taoist belief, a fundamental life force, or Chi, supplies the energy for life. Chi refers both to the breath and to the energies within the body and the surrounding world.

The ancient Taoists, being masters of observation, were able to chart the workings of Chi energy within the human form, as well as in the universe. They mapped the energy field in the human body as a network of channels, or meridians (see pp. 28-9). The unimpeded flow of Chi through the channels was seen as being essential for good health.

Fundamental energy

In Taoist medical practice, Ching Chi, or sexual energy, is the most basic energy in the body and the source of all your energy. By clearing the path of this energy through massage, you can restore the subtle flow of Chi within the channels. In effect, you will be using your sexual energy as a form of medical elixir, to heal illnesses or to increase wellbeing.

Sex and Chinese medicine

A part of Chinese medicine is devoted entirely to sex as a form of healing. A Chinese Taoist physician might well prescribe various sexual techniques, to be practised alone or with a partner, to help treat certain conditions, much as a western physician prescribes drugs. Various physical and emotional disorders would be treated in this way in conjunction with acupuncture and exercise; this makes for a highly enjoyable healing process.

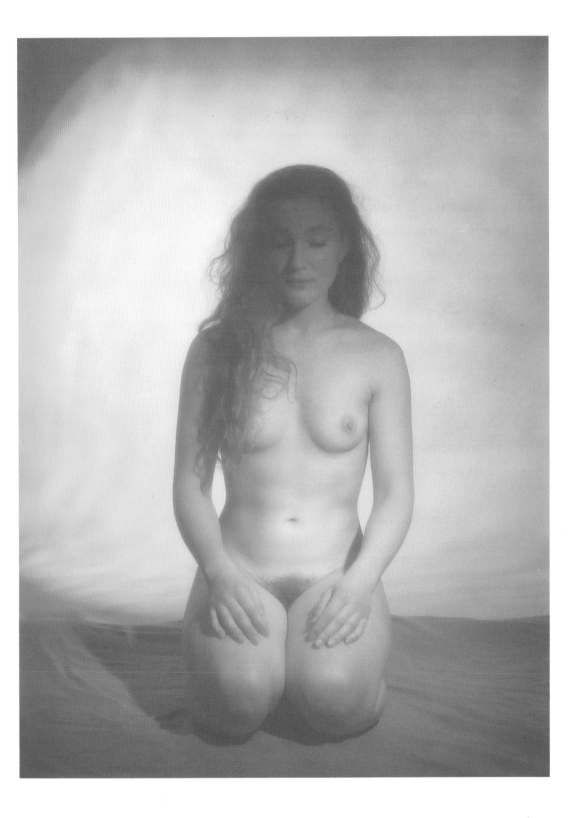

Channels of energy

The twelve channels, or meridians of energy that run through the body, create an endless, interconnecting loop. Both Kirlian photography, which produces an image of the body's electromagnetic field, and methods for testing electrical resistance have recently suggested that such a network of energy exists. But no-one knows exactly how the ancient Taoist sages were able to map the meridians so accurately.

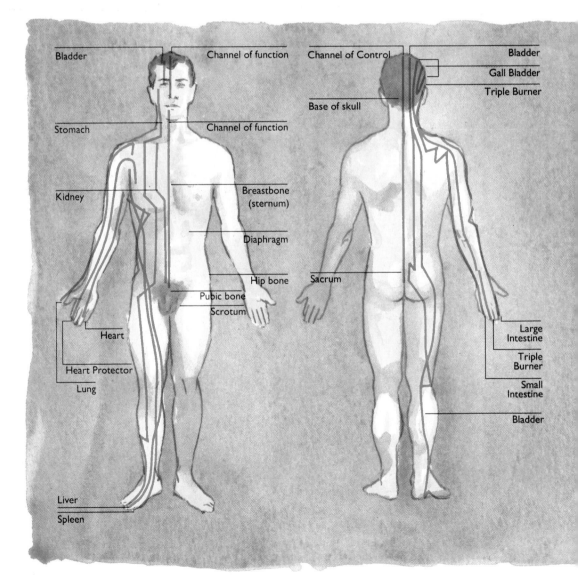

Bladder

Channel of function

Channel of Control

Bladder

Gall Bladder

Triple Burner

Base of skull

Stomach

Channel of function

Kidney

Breastbone
(sternum)

Diaphragm

Hip bone

Sacrum

Pubic bone

Scrotum

Heart

Large
Intestine

Triple
Burner

Heart Protector

Small
Intestine

Lung

Bladder

Liver

Spleen

The complexity and sophistication of the system precludes the development of its form by trial and error. The most respected living Taoist masters say that their predecessors could see the meridians as they observed the patient.

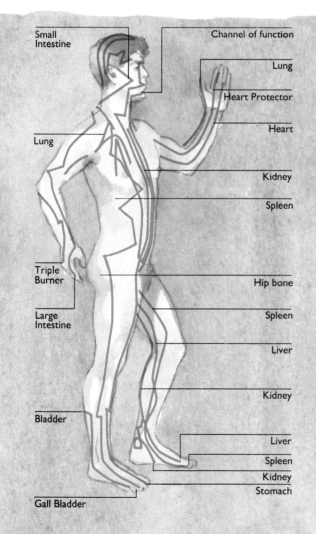

Small Intestine

Channel of function

Lung

Heart Protector

Heart

Lung

Kidney

Spleen

Triple Burner

Hip bone

Large Intestine

Spleen

Liver

Kidney

Bladder

Liver

Spleen

Kidney

Stomach

Gall Bladder

The channel pathways

The energy field
The channels, or meridians, create the energy field of the body. Energy travels in the channels from each of 12 organs, and the channels are linked to make a network. It takes 24 hours for energy to flow through all parts of the network.

The four planes of existence

Sexual energy, the fundamental energy in the body, circulates throughout the energy channels and has an impact on all aspects of our existence. To the Taoist there is no separation between the social, spiritual, mental, and physical planes of existence. They simply represent different levels of energy in the body. From a Taoist viewpoint, the harmony of these four aspects is essential to health. Conflict in the social, mental, spiritual, or physical body manifests as illness.

The aim, the path, and the quest of Taoist sexual practice is to integrate all these aspects of consciousness and the physical functions of the body, to work as a unified being. If you can do this, you can experience a state of ecstasy in all parts of the body together.

Orgasm and spiritual union

In the physical plane, a fully experienced orgasm can free the physical body from muscular rigidity and blocks, allowing blood and nerve energy, or Chi, to circulate freely through the body. At the same time our sexuality is the most obvious path to spiritual union with Creation: in the ecstasy of the fully experienced orgasm we are allowed a short glimpse of the Absolute, or Wu Chi (see right), the ultimate void from which all existence originates, and to where all creation must return. Taoists have since ancient times regarded sexuality as an art, a science, and also a spiritual path. The Chinese Taoist masters considered the feeling of oneness achieved during and following the experience of sexual ecstasy, as being the most easily accessible mystical experience.

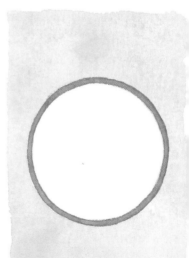

The Wu Chi
Expressed as an empty circle, the Wu Chi is the ultimate void; it represents simultaneously our beginning and our end.

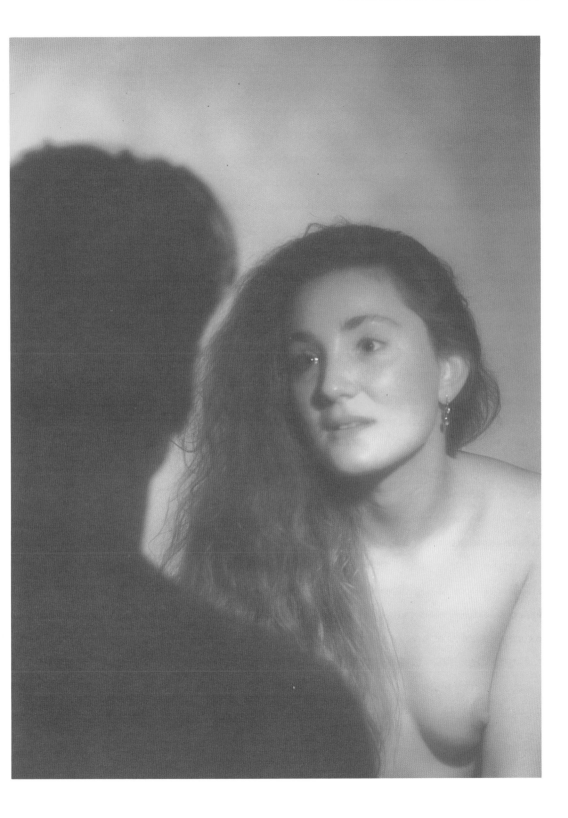

Centres of Divine Energy

Taoist medicine describes the same major energy channels as in classic Chinese medicine, (see pp. 28-9). It explains the way the body functions at a physical and an energetic level. Beyond these exoteric teachings are the esoteric teachings of ancient Taoist sages, which speak of three centres of Divine Energy in the body (see right). These centres are also known as the Tan T'iens, or fields of heavenly elixir.

The role of sexual massage is to ensure the free flow of fundamental sexual energy around the body so that it flows through the Channel of Control and the Channel of Function, and passes through the three centres, or Tan T'iens, linking up and balancing their psychic aspects. In this way, sexuality, courage and passion, intelligence and awareness are all connected (see illustration, right). The Channel of Control (see p. 103) runs upward from the sacrum, along the spinal pathway to the back of the brain. From here it continues as the Channel of Function, over the top of the brain and down again through the middle of the body along the front of the spine, into the perineum.

The most important techniques in the massage sequence (see Part Two) work directly on the Channels of Control and Function; these provide the most direct route for sexual energy from the sacrum up to the brain.

The three Divine Centres

Located in your pelvic abdominal area is the lowest centre. It is here that your sexual energy, vitality, and power are kept and replenished.

The upper abdominal and pectoral region in the centre of the chest is known as the middle Tan T'ien, or middle elixir field. This area stores and regenerates passion, courage, and the powers of communication.

The uppermost Tan T'ien in the mid-brain region is where awareness, including spiritual awareness, and intelligence accumulate and are renewed.

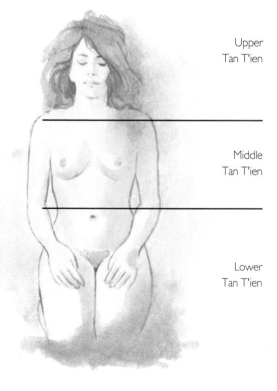

Upper
Tan T'ien

Middle
Tan T'ien

Lower
Tan T'ien

The origin of sexual energy

You inherit your sexual energy from your father and mother at the time of conception. Also known as Ching Chi (see p. 26) or "Ancestral" life energy, sexual energy is the basic force that sustains you throughout life, and when it runs out, you die. The kidneys are responsible for the regeneration of your sexual energy after birth. It is stored in the lower abdomen - the lower Tan T'ien, or Divine Centre (see facing page).

Environmental energy

Sexual energy acts as a catalyst and stimulator for what can be called the environmental Chi energies. These include food, breath, sun, and stimulation energies (see box, right), which circulate throughout the meridian system. Our bodies can only make use of this energy if the flow of fundamental sexual energy is sufficiently strong.

Energy flow and your breathing

Deep, uninhibited breathing keeps this fundamental, sexual energy working at its best. But many of us have lost the habit of breathing freely because of the distortions in our posture and the tension we hold in our bodies. To improve the process of energy circulation, focus on breathing deeply, while imagining the flow of fundamental sexual energy circulating up and down the spine. Take some quiet time every day to practise this simple breathing meditation, and you will enhance your zest and enthusiasm for life, as well as help promote your psychological and emotional wellbeing.

ENVIRONMENTAL ENERGIES

Food energy
Environmental energy obtained from food comes from the nourishment received from the assimilation of nutrients through the digestive tract.

Breath energy
The body's chemical reactions are fuelled on the atomic level from the inhalation and exhalation of air.

Sun energy
Sunlight in its pure form is needed to replenish our psychological and physical energies.

Stimulation energy
Although often overlooked, energy from other external stimuli are also needed for the functioning of human life. Gravity, temperature, air pressure, smell, taste, and even social interaction are some of the major sources of this form of energy.

Circling the sexual energies

Taoist sexual massage produces a strong, free flow of sexual energy circulating throughout your body. This links all planes of existence (see p. 30) and centres of Divine Energy (see p. 32) and, as the sexual energy moves into the upper Tan T'ien, it becomes a creative, spiritual force. A strong circulation of energy also results in glowing vitality and health, increased physical strength, and an ease in manifesting ideas (see p. 38).

Transmuting the sexual energy
As the sexual force moves up to the chest, it infuses the passions. When it reaches the brain, it triggers an altered state of consciousness and a transmutation of sexual energy into a creative, spiritual force (see pp. 30-2).

Circling the sexual energies

Reframing your sexual experience

Many people approach their sexual relationships carrying a burden of expectations based on past experiences. These experiences may be from their own history, or picked up from books, films, or from fantasy. By carrying an image of what it means to be a "good lover", many people believe they have to perform in a certain way during sex. Partners may not take time to settle into the sexual experience, or to become sensitive to the feelings and desires of their partner. Without this care, the sexual act becomes meaningless; at best satisfying the need for the release of tension, at worst leaving both partners feeling frustrated and unsatisfied.

Taoists prefer to shift the goal from good performance or tension release, to finding inner peace and relaxation, calmly enjoying the rise and fall of sexual excitation and sharing that enjoyment with their partner (see below and pp. 56-7). They refine this further by consciously circulating the sexual energy between them (see Achieving the mystical union, p. 36). This leads to a prolonged state of sexual ecstasy, which in turn leads to a heightened state of awareness.

Steps to sexual ecstasy

The first step to achieving a prolonged state of sexual ecstasy is accomplished by reframing your entire sexual experience as a form of meditational practice. The focus shifts from losing yourself in animal abandon, and finally expending all your energy in an uncontrolled orgasm, to staying centred, gently observing the movement of the sexual forces flowing within the bodies during intercourse.

The massage techniques demonstrated in Part Two bring you in touch with the flow of your sexual energy. By learning to observe and control the rise and fall of excitation, you are prepared for a fuller, ecstatic experience during intercourse with your partner.

Achieving the mystical union

When you and your partner learn to reframe your love-making as a meditation (see p. 35), and experience the heightened state of awareness that this brings, you can achieve a mystical union with your own Creation. This is the ultimate goal of Taoist sexual practice. While the massage sequence presented in Part Two is intended to heighten your enjoyment of sexual activities, you can choose whether or not to put it to a more spiritual use. In practice, if you and your partner want to achieve the mystical union of your bodies with the divine creative energies of the universe, you should first follow the Posture Meditation and Navel Breathing Meditation on pages 66-7 and the massage sequence demonstrated in Part Two.

Start with the Posture and Navel Breathing exercises. Once you feel at ease with these techniques, begin the massage sequence (see pp. 94-185) with your partner, taking turns to give and receive. Keep practising the postural and breathing techniques before giving or receiving the massage as well as during the massage itself.

Continue these meditations and the massage for a period of three months, and as you do them, focus on circling the sexual energies throughout your body, as shown on page 34. According to Taoist philosophy, this three month period is sufficient time to strengthen the flow of sexual energy and to familiarize yourself with the techniques before moving on to the next stage.

After three months, you are ready to complete the cycle of male and female energy. During your love-making, whatever position you are in, you can focus on taking your energy upward to your brain, to experience the spiritual effect of your sexual energy. Ideally both of you do this together, although one partner can opt for this change of focus alone.

Breathing slowly, start by drawing the energy up your spine, through the brain, and out through your tongue, to your partner's tongue, from where it travels down your partner's front to the genitals. It is then brought back through your partner's genitals, and the process is reversed.

If the sexual energies of the partners are sufficiently refined, this circling of Divine Energies will draw both partners into spiritual ecstasy, where they will experience a true sharing of spiritual energy and infinite oneness with the divine creative force of the universe. At this point, the sexual aspect is indistinguishable from the spiritual one; the two have merged.

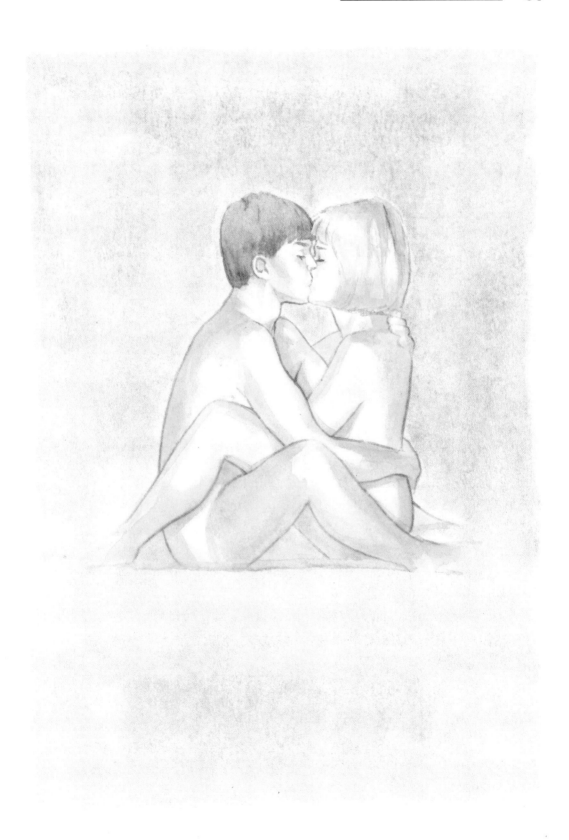

Advanced practice

As a person becomes more proficient in meditative sexual practice, sexual energy becomes more refined, powerful, and easier to channel and direct. This spiritual force of sexual energy reaching the upper Tan T'ien (see p. 32) moves along with the energy in the meridian system of the body and is the same as the energy that flows through the universe.

Whenever you have an idea or intention, such as making something, or travelling somewhere, this idea is projected into the energy system of the universe. The strength and refinement of the energy behind an intention or idea determines the quality and speed with which the idea will be made to happen. At an advanced level of practice, the energy a person is able to project with the ideas will be highly charged, refined, and unhindered in its flow. This means that the manifestation of your aims and wishes occurs with great speed, control, and precision.

As the storehouse of intensified sexual energy develops in the lower abdomen you can use it to fuel the entire body and mind. This storehouse also supplies the energy for the manifestation of ideas into the material plane.

Wu Wei

Wu Wei describes your ability to effect changes in the material world, without making any effort whatsoever. The wisdom of Wu Wei, sometimes translated as "the natural unfolding of events" (see box, right), points out that the best form of action is nonaction - not trying to interfere with this natural course of events - and this is an important psychological preparation for giving and receiving Taoist sexual massage.

The unfolding of events
In Taoist belief, the happenings of the world are unfolding in perfect harmony. In the same way as the unwinding and recombining of the DNA molecule forms new life, the events of the world unfold as conceived by the Divine Law and consciousness of the Tao. If you hold a clear intention of what you are trying to achieve, events will naturally unfold to produce the results you are looking for.

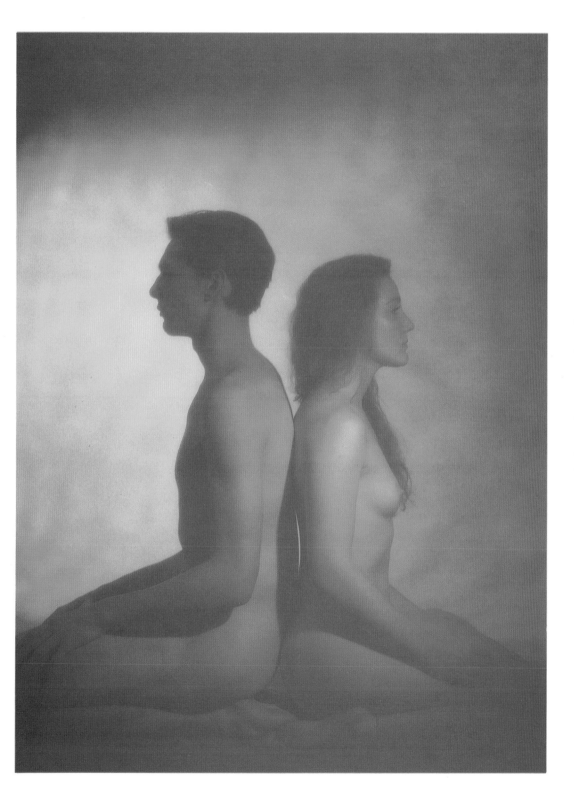

Intention

On a practical level the art of Wu Wei involves the establishment, refinement, and focusing of pure intention for whatever result is desired. In the context of healing, your intention is the most powerful aspect of the art. It overrides all other healing techniques. Pure intention opens the flood gate to allow creative force to enter. The function is more a stepping aside to let happen, than a working hard to achieve. By doing this, you achieve Wu Wei.

However, it would be a fallacy to believe that achieving Wu Wei is the same as doing absolutely nothing. Doing nothing will not automatically fill all your needs and wishes. Just doing nothing creates nothing. To create, you must first prepare a metaphysical space within you that the creative forces can fill (see the Posture Meditation, p. 66). You can do this by relaxation and by becoming one with the Tao. The closer you are to this, the greater will be the wisdom of your intention and the more precious and immediate the results.

As you learn the techniques of sexual massage, take into your practice the notion of Wu Wei; release your tension, and let your body be guided by your healing intent.

Life is light
One of the main obstacles on the path to Wu Wei is seriousness. On the path to oneness with the Tao, seriousness is a form of emotional pestilence. It leads only to constriction and heaviness, and will therefore make your life more arduous than it need be. The path to attainment is built from laughter and lightness of heart. In all that you strive and wish to achieve, it pays to remember, life is light.

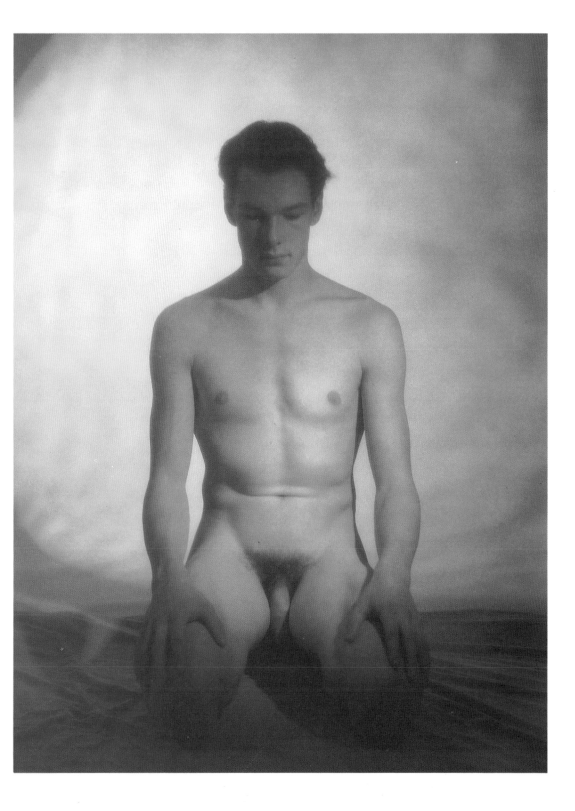

Meditation and ejaculation

For the male, it is the same sexual force that is responsible for the production of semen that is also responsible for the production of general vitality. Adherents of more rigid forms of Taoist practice are not in favour of physical orgasms; they believe that if the practitioner once loses his sperm through ejaculation, he will lose his vitality and will have undone a lifetime of meditative work.

Excessive ejaculation on a regular basis slowly depletes the energy of the kidneys, and so leads to a depletion of overall constitutional strength. This is especially true in the winter months, when the kidneys are more susceptible to cold. However, unnatural suppression of orgasms, which increases the psycho-emotional stress levels, will also deplete the strength of the kidneys.

The more relaxed Taoist practitioners believe that when sperm needs to be released, it will find the way to the surface somehow, and that sperm levels are self-regulating. This second school of thought says that a male must gradually learn to experience a full, uninhibited orgasm. The ultimate aim of learning this is to reach a state of serene detachment at the point of orgasm. This involves the conscious following of the energy backward and upward, rather than forward and outward through the penis (see Circling the sexual energies, p. 34). The energy nourishes the upper Tan T'ien in the brain (see p. 32). Having practised this form of meditation for long enough, a man may be able to experience this peak of excitement without ejaculating. In other words, the emphasis will shift from genital excitation to spiritual excitation.

The true Taoist way of gently, patiently, and lovingly allowing a man to fully enjoy orgasm, until he is able to use the energy to stimulate a spiritual excitation and retain his sperm rather than experience a physical orgasm, has far more long-term value. Needless to say, doing this is a great achievement for the layman.

By contrast, Taoists believe that women gain energy from orgasms. The same mechanism of drawing the explosive sexual energy of the orgasm upward to the brain applies to women. Taoists believe that it is easier for women to achieve this mental focus, as their energy is more Yin, which implies that they are more inward looking, and therefore more in touch with what is going on within them.

By understanding how sexual energy flows throughout your body, and how this energy transmutes into a creative, spiritual force that unites you with the whole of Creation, you can begin to focus on this advanced aspect of Taoist practice. However, whether or not you feel as if you have mastered these advanced practices, you can use the Taoist sexual techniques shown in Part Two of this book to produce an orgasm so sublime and all embracing for both men and women, that union with the supreme Tao is inevitable. This is called the orgasm of the valley, meaning a climax from deep within.

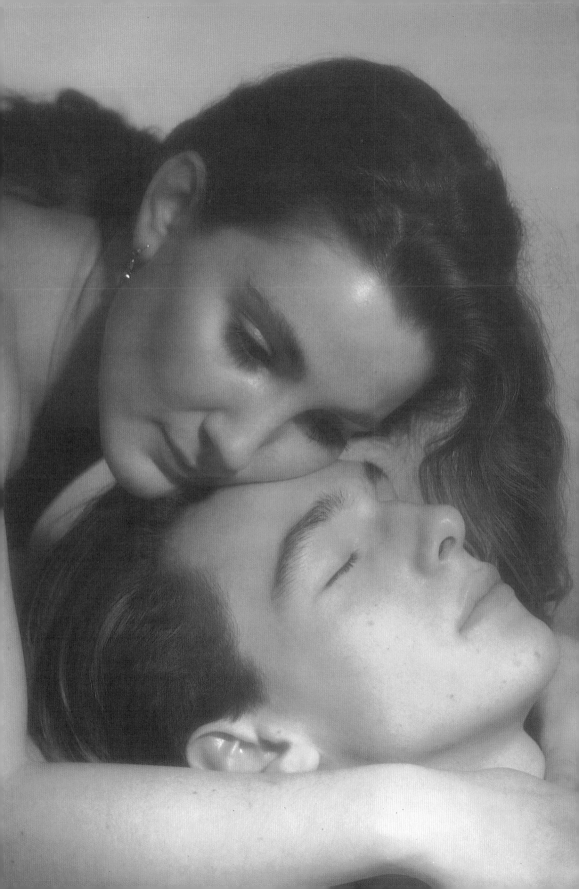

Chapter Two

YOUR SEXUALITY

We are all capable of experiencing great pleasure as children and as adults. We acknowledge such pleasures as eating good food, or enjoying a long walk in the countryside, and actively encourage such pursuits. But we are not taught much about the pleasures that we are able to receive with our bodies, let alone educated in the giving of pleasure to the opposite sex. At best we learn some anatomical facts about the male and female body, but very rarely are we given any insight into the "how to" of body pleasure.

Tension and lack of self-confidence connected with sex and sexuality lead to chronic tension in the body. This restricts the circulation of blood and energy which, in turn, distorts all aspects of the ability to function (see pp. 46-50). In the end, these blocks create obstacles to the full enjoyment of sex and to the ability to enjoy an extended orgasm.

Taoist sexual massage can free the trapped energy produced by your past anguishes, help you to resolve the inner conflicts that surround both your sexuality (see pp. 51-4) and your relationships (see pp. 55-9), and lead you toward a happy, healthy, and fulfilling sexual experience.

THE RELATIONSHIP WITH YOURSELF
Sexuality and pleasure

The ideal start in life for all humans begins with pleasurable sexual intercourse between parents; from these beginnings, the pleasure of your own sexuality should be with you throughout your life. But knowledge of the pleasure that we can experience in ourselves and with others is forbidden for many children. Any restrictions that adults may place on our freedom to explore and enjoy our own sexuality as it emerges will begin to create problems for our sexuality in adolescence and in adulthood.

Children start to become aware of their own sexuality soon after the age of two; from this time they are endowed with an uninhibited, natural sensuousness. But if adults react to this sexuality and sensuality in a negative way, with disregard or shame, it is inevitable that the child will experience an inner conflict about his or her natural feelings, and may interpret this reaction as an unfavourable judgement on their whole being.

Countless generations of humans have been taught, from early infancy on, that touching the genitals is wrong. In a religious context, touching with the aim of inducing pleasure in the genital region was and often still is interpreted as a sin. This emotional conflict between what feels good and yet is at the same time unacceptable will in time lead to guilt and shame. Later these feelings give rise to thoughts of being inferior, or even being fundamentally unclean, which then ignite subconscious thought processes revolving around lack of self worth. In adult life, guilt and shame is further fuelled by the conflict between the search for pleasure, and the constraining forces of social functioning and conditioning.

The effects of guilt and shame are a general loss of love for life, and a rise in the incidence of depression. Your guilt and shame also tend to diminish your appreciation of your own inner beauty, increase the distrust between the sexes, and make you fixate on sexuality as a stimulant.

Everybody affected by feelings of guilt and shame will have negative feelings about their sexuality. These feelings block the flow of primal life force throughout the entire body. Equally, at a physical level, any negativity toward your sexuality or parts of your body leads to chronic tension in muscles throughout the body. This means that your energy can no longer flow between your Tan T'iens, or centres of Divine Energy (see p. 32). The energy in each of these centres becomes trapped. The result is that you are cut off from your deepest sexual feelings.

Taoist sexual and medical practice teaches that for a wholly healthy body and mind, one must fully love and respect the genital region and the sexual force that is harboured there. This positive attitude toward your own sexuality will reflect on the way you treat your child's curiosity and early playful sexual behaviour. In turn your child will emerge into adulthood free of the restrictive blocks that negative behaviour produces.

Blocked energy

The more the natural flow of sexual energy in your body is inhibited, the more it becomes compartmentalized within the three force fields, or Tan T'iens (see p. 47). The Tan T'iens begin to function individually. The energy in the lower force field (see p. 32) - responsible for your sexual energy, vitality, and power - becomes trapped around the genital region. This creates pressure to the point where it can only find release sexually, through the genitals.

In the middle force field, which is located in the chest, the centre of passion, courage, and the powers of communication, the imprisoned energies searching for release will over-stimulate the passion and desires. You will set yourself impossible tasks and generally be over ambitious. The over-stimulated passions can also lead to an unreal, romantic approach to life. The things you hope for can never be realized. Because your desires are out of proportion with what you can achieve, you will lose the harmony in your life.

The energy caught in the upper force field, connected with spiritual awareness and intelligence, leads to over-stimulation of thinking when pressurized. The brain will churn over old programs ad nauseam without resolution of the problems it may be faced with.

Because of the energy blocks, your awareness slides away from the present moment: you no longer focus on the sensations in your body. Your focus will continually shift between an imaginary future, full of hopes and fears, and a distorted past, full of nostalgia and regrets. During sexual activity, this loss of focus on the present moment will cause your attention to wander, and as a result your excitation and generative force will diminish.

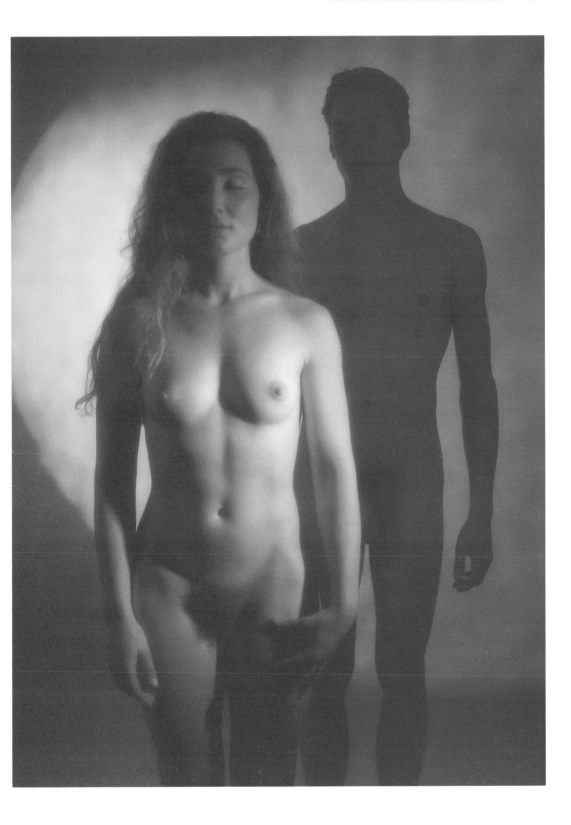

Releasing blocked energy

When the body's energy is compartmentalized (see p. 48), breathing tends to be shallow. Insufficient breathing inhibits the circulation of blood and fluids and creates a band of tension around the upper abdomen and back. It also tenses the diaphragm, which acts like a valve between the Cave of the Original Spirit (the upper Tan T'ien) and the Sea of Vitality (the lower Tan T'ien) (see p. 32 and right).

The key to opening the diaphragm valve is deep, relaxed, breathing (see p. 67). This, and the massage (see Part Two) will open up the pathways of the sexual force, which can then surge up from the lowest Tan T'ien. On its path it will anchor passions and desires and, moving up, enlighten the thought processes, and reunite the three force fields.

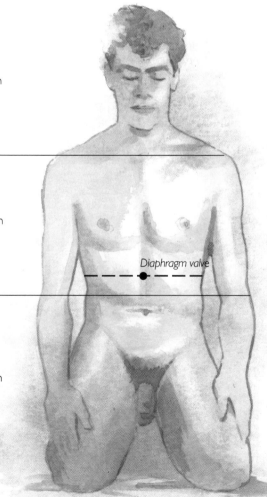

Upper Tan T'ien

Middle Tan T'ien

Diaphragm valve

Lower Tan T'ien

Male and female principle

The most obvious aspect of your sexuality is the sex you are born with. From an early age you are taught by your parents and society what is the scope of acceptable behaviour for a man or a woman. By the time you are adult this programming has permeated your entire being to such an extent that it has become subconscious.

You tend to behave within the limits of your gender role without consciously thinking about your behaviour. For example, as a woman you might automatically think that tools and anything mechanical belong in realm of the male, and so defer the responsibility for repairs to a man; as a man, you might consider the whole issue of child care to be in the domain of the woman and never give this part of existence even the slightest thought.

For the Taoist, all existence stems from the interplay of Yin and Yang, so it follows that the differences between body and mind of man and woman are just seen as a natural continuation of the Yin and Yang cosmology (see pp. 22-3). However, Taoism has for thousands of years acknowledged something that western science has only recently confirmed. Biologically, the polarity of gender continues all the way down to cellular level. And the delicate balance of male and female hormones within the body determines the sexual identity of a person.

Anima and Animus

It was the psychologist Carl Jung who introduced the idea that this biological fact has its counterpart in the psyche. Jung claimed that within the psyche of the man resided a female element, which he called Anima. Likewise he assumed a male element, Animus, within the psyche of woman.

For the Taoist the biological and the psychological truth of this has been known since the formulation of the Yin Yang theory. Taoists maintain that in each person, man or woman, both Yin and Yang energies are contained. The interplay between them sustains the psychological and biological life of the individual.

Worldly existence depends on these two forces. Enlightenment, or becoming one with the Tao, requires the harmonization of male and female principles within you to the point where they merge and become one. To achieve this a person must strive to integrate the male and female polarities. On the psychological level this can be done by exploring the nature of our inner opposites (see box, below).

Your lover as your inner opposite

The key to exploring your inner opposite is in understanding that the woman or man you are living with, or attracted to, is likely to be very much like your internal opposite. This choice represents your divine essence striving to achieve oneness with the Tao from your very beginning. Understanding this principle profoundly alters the quality of relating to the opposite sex.

Reflected behaviour

Whatever your view is toward the opposite sex, it will be reflected upon the inner male or female within you. Whatever actions you take toward the opposite sex, whether good, bad, or indifferent, you will be doing the same to your inner opposite self. Even if the wisdom of this escapes you for the moment, it pays for you to treat your lover as if they are the divine projection of your inner opposite.

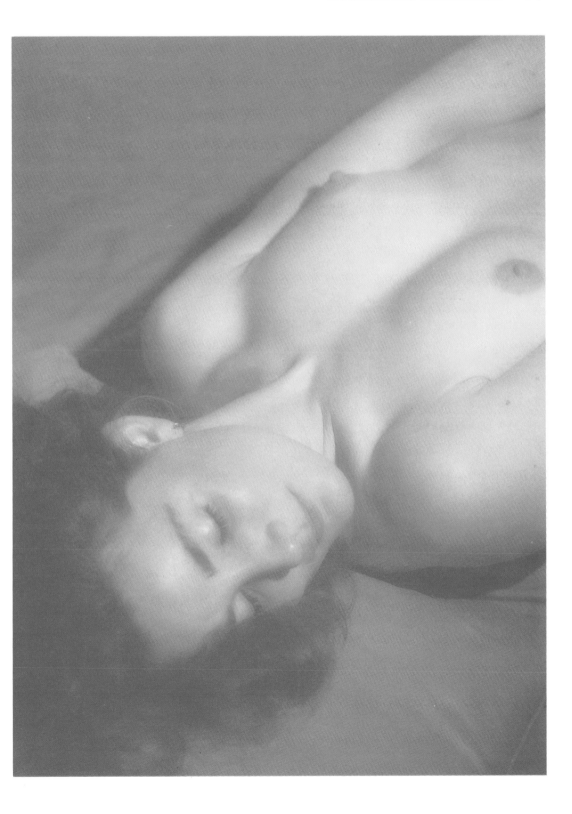

Self love, self massage, and masturbation

Before it is possible to love another person, we must learn to love ourselves, not in a self indulgent way, but to experience love as a positive feeling toward ourselves and our bodies.

The first step on the path to self love is bodily self acceptance. Negative self judgements of the body create internal conflict, which lead to low self esteem and can disrupt the flow of Chi through the body (see pp. 46-7). Any massage, especially a sexual massage, helps to balance your attitude toward your body. The very application of healing touch to your body affirms of your self worth and self love.

If you have no partner with whom to exchange a sexual massage, try massaging yourself. Getting to know your body through your own touch not only relieves minor aches and pains by eliminating toxins from the tissue, but connects your energy circuits, freeing the flow of Chi. Any of the techniques described in this book can be used for self massage, providing that they are within reach. Vary the massage to suit your needs. Treat every part of your body with respect, and aim to give yourself the utmost pleasure.

If you automatically shy away from areas of your body, this indicates that you are unconsciously separating yourself from them, which restricts the flow of Chi. Continue to massage these parts gently, to help to reintegrate them and re-establish energy flow. If your self massage leads to masturbation, reassure yourself that even though it cannot create the same circulation of energies as between two individuals (see pp. 36-7), it will help to soothe away some of your energy blocks.

YOUR RELATIONSHIP WITH OTHERS
Puritanism and hedonism

We come to relationships full of expectations of how our partner should behave toward us, and how we should feel and behave toward our partner. When these expectations are not met we become frustrated and angry. This anger creates tension in the body, which causes blocks in the sexual energy flow (see p. 48). Often the two partners do not share the same desires, needs, or expectations of each other, and the stress created by this imbalance can also block the sexual energy flow.

In Taoist thinking sexual blocking can manifest as one of two extremes - a puritanical suppression of sexual urges or a hedonistic craving for sex at any cost.

Puritanism and hedonism are like Yin and Yang - two sides of a dichotomy. Without the fear of unbridled, individual lust and pleasure, puritanism cannot exist. In contrast puritanism, by its negation of the fundamental necessity for eroticism, and because of its strict moral views, creates the knee-jerk reaction of hedonism.

Puritanism and self censorship
Many people in the West adopt a puritanical attitude toward sexuality, consciously controlling and regulating sexual desire and passion, subconsciously suppressing natural animal urges. Many decisions in a puritanical way of life are to a very large extent subconscious. The puritanical attitude is frequently kept alive by a constant internal dialogue, a little like a censorship committee guiding the thought processes. This committee is continually giving value judgements about behaviour. In time this encourages a state of neurotic and

unnecessary tension in the body, mind, and spirit, blocking
the flow of sexual energy (see p. 48). Although this may
serve to protect people from disharmony in their personal
lives, it does so at the expense of natural, physical joy.

Hedonism

The hedonistic attitude toward sexuality - consciously seeking
out physical pleasure and self expression for its own sake,
and allowing lust or desire to lead you headlong and
unconsciously into doing things you may afterwards regret -
eventually leads to a feeling of unfulfilment, and to a life that
is devoid of true meaning.

Although pleasure can relax the body temporarily, and
lend some colour to thought processes, it will do so at the
expense of true inner depth and peace.

In its extreme form, hedonism can be socially disruptive
and will create a person who is lonely, and unable to sustain
intimacy and form and maintain authentic relationships.

The Taoist middle path

There is however a third choice, which is to adopt a Taoist
attitude, and frame the entire encyclopedia of sexual
experience in the context of a meditation (see p. 35).

Once embraced, it is possible to sit in the midst of
events, serenely observing the rise and fall of desire and
excitation. The key to being able to do this is to make
yourself aware of, and then suspend, all self judgement or
self congratulation toward sexual experiences. Now pleasure
is no longer good or bad, it is simply an experience of
energy. In the same way, deprivation of pleasure no longer
has a value attached, it now simply "is". Using this technique
of suspended judgement, both pleasure and lack of it are
brought back under control. The occurrence of sexual energy

is observed, but no longer gives rise to an automatic response.

For most people, sexual energies are experienced with such force that there seems no alternative but to react to them. Essentially this is because a value (e.g. good or bad, nice or disturbing) is attached to the rising feeling. Along with a value we tend to give rising energetic feelings a name. For example you might experience a tickling feeling in the genital region, to which you will then, usually without conscious thought, attach a value and a name (e.g. sexual excitement). This unconscious naming and valuing then triggers chain reactions in the thought processes. You might think to yourself "what an inopportune time to have sexual feelings", or you might make a date for later on. Whatever the thoughts generated, they will have taken you away from the original feeling. The Taoist way is simply to put awareness into the feeling - to observe yourself fully experiencing the feeling without either valuing or naming it. This conscious observation transforms your experience of the feeling from a hedonistic to a spiritual one. The exercise (right) will help you practise this technique. Ultimately the aim is to observe, enjoy, and let pass, as all states eventually do.

Naturally this technique is not learned overnight. Like most skills it will take time to achieve mastery. A beginner might find it impossible to stay focused for longer than a few seconds, or that the urge for sexual gratification is too strong not to be followed. This is natural, and should be expected. When practising directing your awareness, be easy on yourself. The trick, as in all of the techniques in this book, is to relax, and to concentrate on your breathing.

In following the Taoist path there is no failing. Even if you can only focus for a short period on your feelings without your mind interfering, it will help to sweeten your sexual experience.

*Directing awareness
to the feeling*
Sit or lie comfortably. Take three deep, slow breaths. Now, mentally isolate the area of your solar plexus - the diaphragm. Using muscular force, tense the area as much as you can for about 3 seconds. Now relax and breathe. Repeat this twice. Now place your awareness into the area with concentration by directing your mind to what you are feeling. Feel whether it is hot or cold, tight or loose.

Allow the tone of this feeling to expand, until it fills your whole body and finally disappears.

Longstanding relationships

In an ideal world, you are attracted to your partner so strongly that this excludes desire or lust for another person for the rest of your life. However, in the real world, there is hardly a person that has not, even if only in the mind, been unfaithful to their companion or spouse at one time or another. We may think that just having unfaithful thoughts has nothing to do with bodily unfaithfulness, but for your divine inner core there is no difference whatsoever. To know this leaves the majority of us in a dilemma. To stay faithful to your partner all the way down to your divine inner core is, under these circumstances, impossible.

In some ways, faithfulness is contrary to the natural flow of life. The reason for this is that faithfulness or fidelity is basically a social function. It is generally definable as the repression of the sexual urge in order to further the ideal of the couple, the smallest social unit possible.

Here again we meet the conflict between what is experienced as being pleasurable - bringing a sparkle to the eye - and what is in the view of society or your partner, unacceptable (see also p. 46). Such a conflict will lead to guilt and shame. The partner who responds to the urge for sexual gratification outside of the relationship may feel that he or she has betrayed trust, which will lead to conscious or subconscious feelings of guilt and shame and from there to resentment toward the other partner. The same will happen even if one or both of the partners in a relationship are experiencing yearnings to have sexual experiences with other people, but out of loyalty or fear do not respond to them. In this case the tendency is for the partner who is denying the urge subconsciously to make the other responsible for the losing out on pleasure. As before, this will lead to resentment.

The betrayed partner usually experiences jealousy. To understand jealousy we must realize that it is typically the many faceted experience of the fear of abandonment or loss. Since fear is intimately connected to survival, jealousy can sometimes take on forms and proportions beyond anything that any person can logically explain. This is due to an actual physical hormonal release of adrenalin (kidney energy) in response to what is subconsciously perceived as a threat. As neither jealousy or resentment is functional to a relationship, they need to be resolved.

The idea that fidelity is the same thing as sexual faithfulness is a misconception. It stems from the belief that the sexual force is the underlying principle of the relationship between partners. From a spiritual Taoist point of view, however, faithfulness is a condition of the heart and the divine inner spirit, and not of the sexual organs. The function of sexuality is to be creative, the function of the heart is to be connected. If you make your relationship a spiritual search for oneness, you can harness the creative forces of sexuality within your relationship, and achieve oneness with the Tao, which is indistinguishable from oneness with your partner. Even if only briefly experienced, this state will reveal the true meaning of faithfulness, and sexuality will from then on be seen as the tool that it actually represents.

Seeing the divine inner spirit
Every day remind yourself to look for the connectedness of all phenomena, people, and events. Disregard all thoughts of separateness and in time you will see the spirit shining through your partner's eyes. This regenerates feelings of tenderness and caring within your relationship.

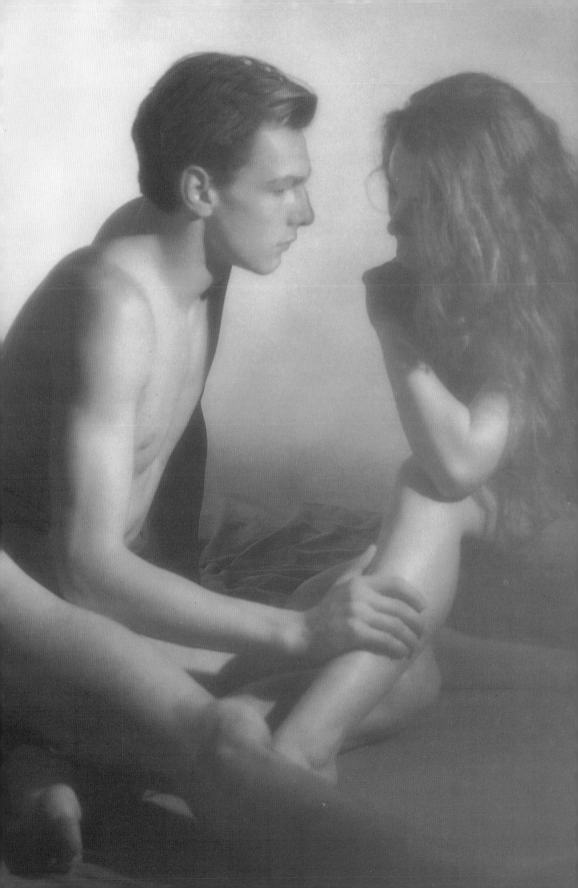

Chapter Three

PREPARING YOURSELF

BEFORE starting the massage sequence it is essential to prepare the physical space around you and to create the right state of mind, or mind-set, for both giver and receiver. This will determine the success of the massage for both partners; if it starts with one or both of you feeling nervous, tense, or angry, this feeling will detract from the experience.

To prepare the physical space, make the room feel comfortable and secure (see p. 62) and choose your massage oil (see pp. 63-4). To create your mental space, start by letting your partner know in advance that you would like to do a sexual massage; the preparation for a massage actually begins at this time of setting the intention. This does not, however, exclude you from doing the massage in a spontaneous fashion.

To give or receive the massage you need to let your mind move into a trance-type state to heighten your sensations (see p. 65). The Posture Meditation and Navel Breathing Meditation exercises (see pp. 66-7) are important for achieving this alteration in consciousness. Practise them before beginning to learn the massage sequence in Part Two; subsequently, continue to use them as preparation every time you start the massage.

PREPARING THE PHYSICAL SPACE
Comfort and security

It pays to take time in advance to prepare the room you will be using. There is nothing more annoying than having to break the continuity of the massage because you have to get oil or search for another towel, cushion, condom, or something to drink. If both partners are to give the massage in turn, prepare the massage space together; this also gives time to settle in.

Make sure that the room is warm, private, and secure. A cotton mattress, such as a Japanese-style futon, or layers of blankets placed on the floor make a good massage surface. It is possible to use a standard massage table, but this does not allow as much direct contact between partners as does working on the floor. If you use oil (see facing page), warm it before beginning the massage (see p. 64), and have it at hand. Keep the room warm, too, and offer your partner a large towel or soft blanket to maintain a comfortable temperature over the parts of your partner's body that you are not working on. A small cushion and a second blanket also help to make the receiver more comfortable (see p. 71).

To make this a real celebration of sex and eroticism, beautify and sensualize the room with flowers; burn some incense and decorate the space with any good luck charms or objects that have a spiritual value for you. You might also consider taking a bath or shower together before the start of the massage. This is a wonderful way to make a break in the everyday flow of life, and will make both giver and receiver feel relaxed, clean, and secure.

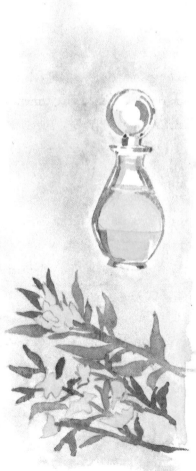

Using oils

Massage oil allows your hands to glide easily and sensuously over your partner's body without creating friction. It also nourishes the skin. Choose between scented and unscented oils. For unscented oil, vegetable oil such as sunflower, safflower, or grapeseed oil will do perfectly well. Olive oil tends to be too thick. Mineral oil such as baby oil is only a second best choice, as it is not easily absorbed by the skin.

You may find that scented oils have an even more pleasing effect. There is a strong relationship between smells and sexual excitement, which is in part due to the fact that some perfumes contain substances that mimic the smell of human sexual hormones and pheromones (message-laden substances secreted by your glands). Musk, which smells like the male sexual hormone testosterone, is the most well known of these. Scented oils have been used since antiquity for rituals of sexual excitement and pleasure. They will enchant both giver and receiver of a massage.

Making your own, unique, perfumed massage oil is easy, fun, and much cheaper than buying it ready made. As a base, any of the above-mentioned vegetable oils will do. Add a few drops of perfume or essential oil for a distinct scent and properties. Aphrodisia oil (see recipe, right) is popular for use with the sexual massage sequence.

Smell is a very personal issue. Experiment with essential oils until you find a smell to your liking. Try Rose, Musk (see above), Ylang Ylang, Orchid, Vanilla, or Cinnamon scents, all of which are beneficial and complement the Taoist massage technique.

Once you have created your oil, store the preparation in

Recipe for Aphrodisia oil
To make this sensuously stimulating massage oil, start by mixing 60ml (2 fl oz) Sweet Almond oil with 5ml (1 teaspoon) Jojoba oil. Add to the mixture 6 drops of Wild Musk oil, 4 drops of Rose oil, and 3 drops of Rosewood oil. Mix thoroughly. This makes enough for several massages.

an airtight container in the refrigerator. Oil that is warm and
exposed to air will rapidly oxidize, turn rancid, and become
unusable. Before starting a massage, warm the oil by placing
the container in hot water.

Quantity

Sensuous massage especially requires a gentle touch; too
much oil makes close contact with your partner's skin
impossible and the overall effect will not be pleasing. Pour
about half to one teaspoonful of oil into your palm. Rub
your palms together to spread the oil and to warm your
hands before starting the massage. Reapply it as often as you
need during the massage to keep your hands lubricated.

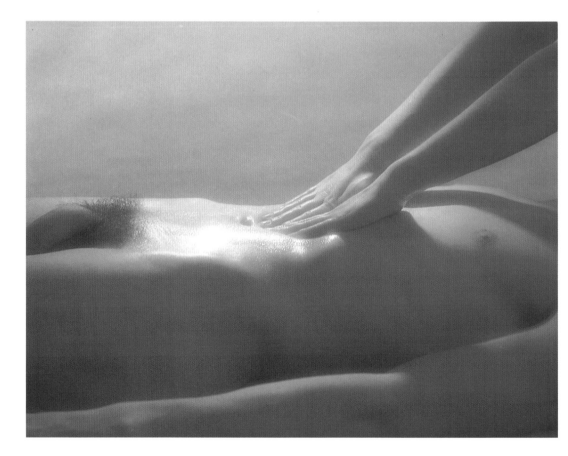

PREPARING YOUR MENTAL SPACE
Altered states

In daily life, we take in information using our five senses - by seeing, hearing, feeling, smelling, and tasting. The eyes provide the primary source of information for most people; we are constantly analyzing and responding to visual information. But to make a sexual massage work, the giver and the receiver must shift from the visual to a feeling mode of being, in which the sense of touch is heightened. Confining your awareness to the feeling mode heightens your focus; this change in awareness is called a trance. It is this trance state that you are aiming to achieve when giving or receiving a sexual massage.

Meditations for shifting the awareness

Practise the following posture and breathing meditations before you start to learn the massage sequence, and as a preparation for giving or receiving a sexual massage.

Continued practice - whether on your own or with your partner - enables you to develop and circulate a storehouse of energy. It brings inner peace, and a sharper mental focus as well as improved blood circulation.

As you practise, make a mental picture of the upper, middle, and lower centres (see p. 32). Visualize and focus on those parts of the body you are working on (see p. 57).

Making an agreement
If you are doing this massage with someone for the first time, we suggest that you agree upon a contract of conduct. This gives you the opportunity to talk over such matters as taking or not taking turns as giver and receiver (see p. 93), having or not having sex, and so forth. It is also the time to discuss contraception and the issue of using condoms for the prevention of sexually transmitted diseases.

Massage and meditation
These breathing and postural changes move you into a meditative state that prepares you for giving or receiving a sexual massage, able to respond fully to your partner, yet collected enough to enjoy the process of the massage as a form of meditation (see pp. 35 and 56-7).

Posture Meditation

This basic preparation for opening up the body's energy pathways changes your level of awareness and heightens the sense of touch throughout the massage. Take a few deep breaths to help quieten your mind. Practise this technique alone or with your partner until you are accustomed to how it feels. Then you will be able to keep your back lengthened and widened while giving and receiving the massage.

Anchoring your spine

Feel and visualize your spine firmly anchored at the sacrum by its connection to the hips. This anchor gives stability to the structure. Remember that your spine is the axis and support for the entire physical structure of your body.

Lengthening your spine

In visualizing your spine, think of your entire skull as the uppermost vertebra, which just happens to be enlarged enough to house your brain and support your face. Feel as if your skull, this top-most "vertebra", is floating upward like a balloon. This has the effect of lengthening your spinal column.

With your mental focus alone, without stretching or straining, picture your entire spinal column firmly anchored at the hips and lengthening upward.

Widening your torso

Once you are comfortable with this image of your spine and the sensation that ensues, you can begin to imagine and feel your entire torso and head broadening out sideways.

Start this by picturing your sitting and hip bones broadening, moving further away from each other sideways. Then, while still holding the image of your lengthening spine, picture your middle and upper back broadening so that your shoulder blades feel as if they are moving away from each other. Finally, feel the back of your head becoming broader, so that your ears seem to be moving further apart from each other.

You will begin to feel that you are metaphysically occupying more space even though you are physically no larger. Follow this metaphysical space meditation with the Navel Breathing Meditation exercise (see facing page).

Navel Breathing Meditation

The Navel Breathing Meditation is the second part of the exercise for changing your awareness to a feeling mode. It works on the rhythm of your breath, so that your body's energy shifts from your head to the centre of your body. Your breathing enables you to harness your mental focus and use this to send sexual energy around your body.

The natural breath

Picture a sponge inside your lower abdomen, below the navel, that soaks up air instead of water. First, you must squeeze it empty. Gently pull in the muscles of your abdomen to their natural limit without straining, until the sponge is empty. Then gently release the abdominal muscles; this allows the sponge to expand and soak up air again as you inhale. As the breath rushes in, your abdomen will visibly expand. As soon as the sponge is filled with air, pull in the abdominal muscles once again to squeeze the sponge and exhale to release the air.

Once you are comfortable with this basic, natural breathing mechanism, begin to integrate it with the Meditation Posture (see facing page).

Integrated meditation

As breath enters your body, focus your attention on your broadening hips, torso, and head.

As breath leaves your body, focus your attention on your lengthening spine.

It can take many years or just one second to understand, assimilate, and perform the merging of these two meditations. Once mastered and practised with regularity, you will be able to use it with ease to assist the flow of energy while you give or receive the massage.

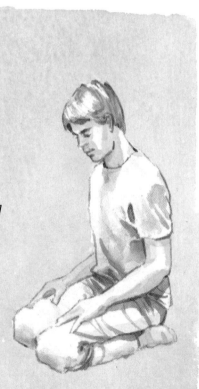

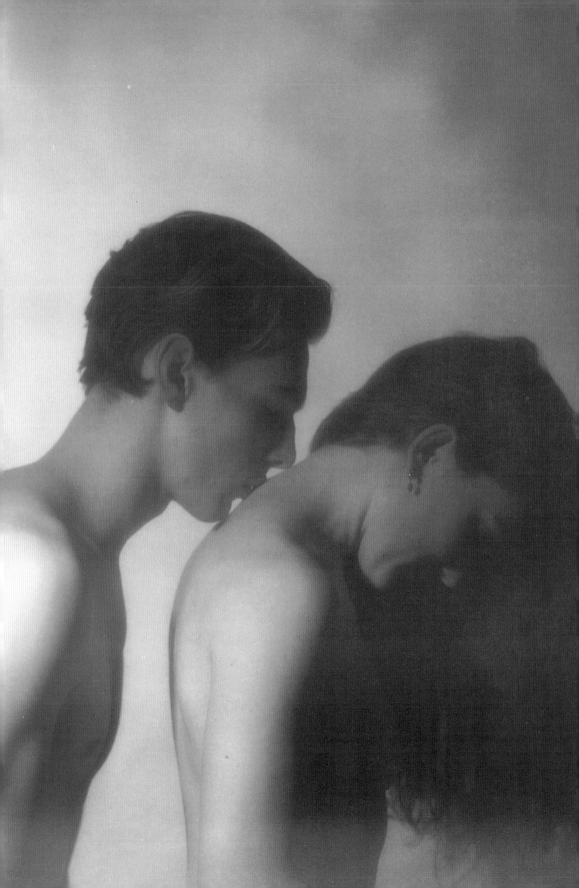

Chapter Four

BEFORE YOU BEGIN

ONCE you have prepared your mental and physical space, and
practised the Posture and Navel Breathing Meditations (see Chapter
Three), you are almost ready to begin the massage sequence.

This chapter introduces you to the roles of giver and
receiver, and to the most comfortable positions to take up during
the massage (see pp. 70-4). The hand techniques are described on
pages 77-83, with a discussion of their healing energy on pages 75-6.
The basic hand positions and the four basic strokes you need for the
massage are described on pages 77-83.

The massage moves energy through the body and follows the
course outlined on page 84. While there are no rules about performing the massage in a particular order, it is a useful way to learn.

Within the sequence of the massage are resting positions,
and moments where the contact between giver and receiver is
broken altogether. These have their own part to play in the
massage, as described on page 86. A note on the timing of the
massage sequence (see p. 88) concludes the chapter, with a
reassuring note that, as with all Taoist text, the instructions given
are intended as no more than helpful suggestions to maximize
your enjoyment.

The receiver

To receive a sexual massage requires nothing more from you than to be willing to accept and enjoy the pleasure that your partner gives you. Your ability to give up control to your partner during the massage will to a large extent govern your capacity to receive pleasure. Be ready to accept the form, or pattern, that the massage takes. This does not mean that you have to continue with the massage if any aspect of it disagrees with you. Reserve the right to say "stop", at any time, if you feel the need to.

Bear in mind that this massage is designed to raise your tolerance for ecstatic, or blissful experiences. For some people, bliss is as hard to bear as pain is for others. If you feel that you belong to the group of people with a low bliss tolerance level, use this massage as an opportunity to expand your limits. It may take time to learn to accept this level of pleasure. Whatever you do, always remember to enjoy your body.

Position of receiver

When receiving a massage, your partner should maintain a lengthened and relaxed spine. The Posture Meditation on page 66 is a useful preparation for this.

For the first part of the massage - the Preparation Sequence (pp. 94-9) and for the Front Sequence (pp. 132-84), your partner lies face up. In order to remain comfortable and relaxed, and maintain a lengthened and relaxed spine, it may help to place a rolled blanket under the backs of the knees, and to place a small pillow under the head.

Make sure that your partner's legs are lying straight, not crossed, and that they are symmetrically placed. Check that the body is straight, head aligned with the legs.

For the Back Sequence (see pp. 100-29), when the receiver is lying face down, it is advisable to place a rolled blanket under the shins. This raises the feet and so takes the strain off the knees.

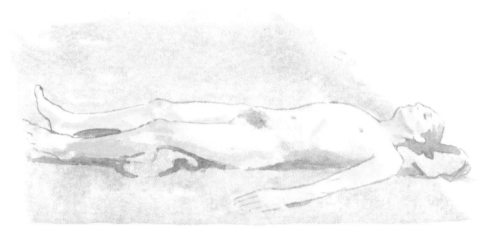

Using blankets for comfort

When lying on your back, roll a small blanket and place it under the knees to keep the spine relaxed. Use a small pillow under the head (see below, top).

When lying on your front, use a rolled blanket under the shins to take strain off the knees (see below, bottom).

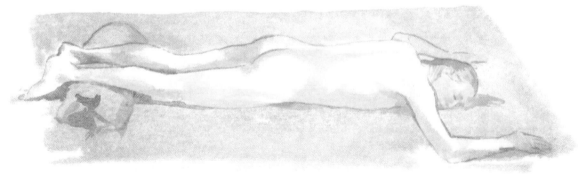

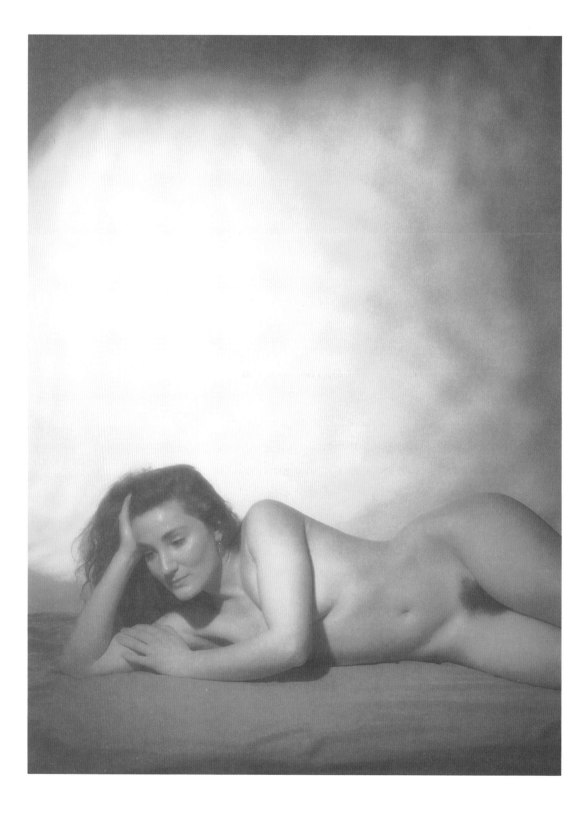

The giver

As a giver, do your best to rid your mind of all thoughts concerning your own sexual gratification. Dedicate yourself to healing and empty your mind so that you can be a vessel for the healing energy of the Tao, using the therapeutic touch of your hands. Set your intention on purely serving, healing, and giving pleasure. To give a sexual massage requires you to be soft and natural.

Whether sitting on your heels, or squatting upright, elongate your spine and relax your shoulders. Keep your breathing, slow, deep, and regulated. No strain or great energy expenditure is required. You need only enough strength to maintain the form of your hands and arms (see the four basic hand positions, pp. 77-82). The more you relax within your body, the more the healing and harmonizing energies of the Tao can flow through you, out through your palms and into your partner.

Make sure that the point from which you move, and all your hand movements, are instigated by the energy in the lower abdomen. Let the hands merely be instruments, the Tao is the player. Almost all of the sequence requires a flowing, feather-light touch, as if skimming your palms over water. By moving your hands lightly in this way over the various channel pathways (as shown in Part Two), you will direct the flow of subtle energies toward the sexual centre. As you do this, your partner may experience a heightened sensual enjoyment in the lower abdomen and genitals. If you feel yourself or your partner becoming too excited, stop, and place your hands in one of the resting positions (see p. 86) to settle the energy and pull your partner back from the acceleration of sexual force. Synchronize your breathing patterns with your partner to assist the calming process. Keep your awareness in your hands, then start to inhale and exhale in unison with your partner. Although this may seem to be a very simple technique, the results may well surprise you. When you and your partner feel more calm and centred, take up the massage sequence again, moving the sexual energy.

As you lead your partner through rising and falling excitation levels (see pp. 84-5), she or he may begin to experience a strongly altered state of mind. When properly performed the massage orchestrates the force of sexual energy to a point where your partner will feel complete and nurtured.

Position of giver

During much of the sequence, you will be sitting on your heels. You may find that your knees and feet ache at first. If so place a folded blanket between your buttocks and your heels.

Always focus on your spine feeling lengthened, your torso and head broadened, and your spine firmly anchored at the hips (see p. 66).

Keep your upper back and chest open and broad, your shoulders relaxed, and your armpits empty of tension.

Magnetic healing energy of the hands

By moving from your lower abdomen, using your energy from your own inner centre, your hands will become like "energy magnets". Holding your palms a little above your partner's skin, you will be effecting a magnetic pull. Whenever you place your hands on your partner's body, you will draw all similar energies into that part of the body. You can use this magnetic pull for healing and harmonizing purposes.

The most advanced practitioners of Taoist medicine maintain that they can diagnose and heal patients using the magnetic energies of their hands alone. Some highly developed masters of this art assert that they need no actual physical contact to achieve this. Within Taoist medicine, physicians with the ability to use the magnetic healing force of the hands for therapeutic intervention are highly valued. This method of treatment is considered to be the most superior form of therapy, and is believed to be more effective than acupuncture, or the use of herbs, since it involves the direct manipulation of the flow of fundamental energy.

Unless you belong to this group of exceptional medical master physicians, you would be ill-advised to expect to be able to manipulate the fundamental energies of the body enough to facilitate lasting fundamental changes in the body's energy flow. In practice, this means that you cannot hope to heal a seriously ill person; such fundamental changes can only be produced by master physicians.

Nevertheless, everyone has the ability to utilize the healing magnetic qualities of their hands to a certain extent. Everyone is able to use their hands to draw energy to various parts of the body. All that is needed is simple laying-on of

hands in a meditative way, using the healing commands that
are given below (see box, left).

It is said that those people who proceed through life
aiming to achieve oneness with the Tao, and hence oneness
with themselves, will become more and more able to
influence and harmonize energies with the magnetic healing
force of their hands.

Healing commands

*Within Taoist medical philosophy,
a headache can be caused by an
excessive build up of "heat energy"
within the head. If you place your
right hand with a command "hot"
on the suffering person's sacrum,
you will soon feel heat building up
under the palm of your hand. If
you leave it there for a while to
grow hotter and hotter, by the
power of your mind and energy
alone, it will attract all the heat
from the head. This in turn will
help clear the headache. To further
assist the healing process you can
then place your left hand with the
command "cool" on the forehead.
This will attract cooling energies to
the forehead, which will further
clear the symptoms.*

Feeling the magnet powers

*The following exercise is designed
for you to experience the magnetic
power of your palms. Hold your
hands out in front of you, palms
facing each other, two inches (5cm)
apart. With shoulders relaxed, move
your palms away from each other
and back again, as if squeezing a
concertina. After a while, as you
concentrate on the centre of each
palm, you will feel the magnetic
pull between your palms. The
amount of pull will be different for
each person. Time of day, emotional
stability, physical strength, and the
overall balance of energies within
your body all influence the
magnetic pull of your hands.*

THE FOUR BASIC HAND POSITIONS

Four basic hand positions enable you to perform the whole massage sequence (see pp. 94-184). Each has a different effect on your partner's energy (see p. 78). But whichever you use - percussion (see p. 78), the Flat Hand Stroke (see p. 80), the One Finger Stroke (see p. 81), or the Pulling Stroke (see p. 82) - keep hands and fingers relaxed and soft, but remember that the shape must always be definite.

Use a light touch (see box, right). While there will be times when your intuition will guide you to press more firmly, you should tease and beckon the energy, never force it.

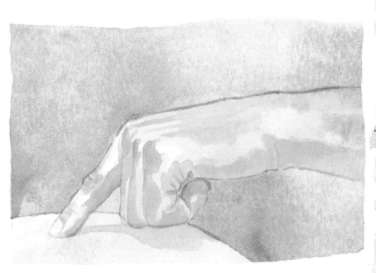

Using a light touch

During a sexual massage you are dealing primarily with energy in the body, not only the physical form. Generally, the lighter your touch, the more powerful the response you will elicit. Masters of this art can effect the greatest results by running their hands just above the physical body (see p.75).

Percussion

Percussion is a stimulating form of massage stroke (see below). Loosely clench your fists and then, using alternate hands, let them fall repeatedly and rhythmically on to the area you are massaging. Begin by trying out this technique on a pillow, on your own leg, or on any other soft surface. It is easy to be heavy handed with your fists, but by practising in this way you can learn to keep the strokes light. Keep your hands relaxed while performing the strokes. This lets your fists bounce, making it easy to sustain a rhythmic change of hands.

Energy from your strokes

Percussion is used for vigorous stimulation of energy and has the advantage of working quickly. The receiver can feel the effects immediately, usually as a fizzing sensation produced by energy below the area that you are working on.

The body responds instantly to percussion. The rhythm is like an echo of the mother's heart beat, heard before birth. It is the same as the body's response to the beat of tribal drums or to the computerized beat of a modern dance record. The external response to rhythmic percussion in a dancer indicates the extent of the internal energy response in the person receiving the percussion stroke in massage.

The Flat Hand Stroke (see p. 80) is used to push energy along the pathway - like a swimmer pushing through water while doing breast stroke.

The One Finger Stroke (see p. 81) is used to tease energy along when more subtle manipulation is required. It is like rolling a fine, round pearl along under the fingertip.

The Pulling Stroke (see p. 82) is used for the same energetic result as the Flat Hand Stroke. It is like pulling silk from a cocoon.

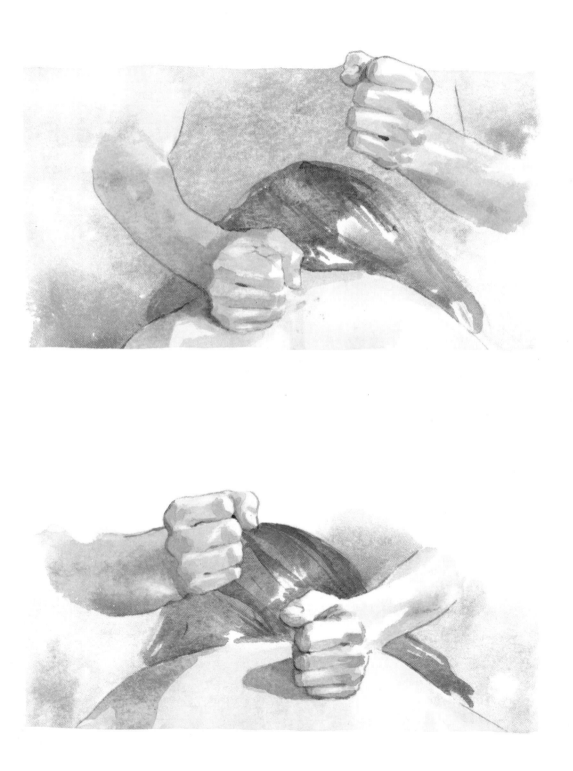

The Flat Hand Stroke

In this position the hand is held with the fingers pulled up, almost into a bow shape (see illustration, below).

Use the middle section of the fingers, just below the distal joint, to guide the direction of the palm. Apply pressure through the mounds that lie below the base of the fingers, at the top of the palm. Let your hand be sensitive to the contours of your partner's skin.

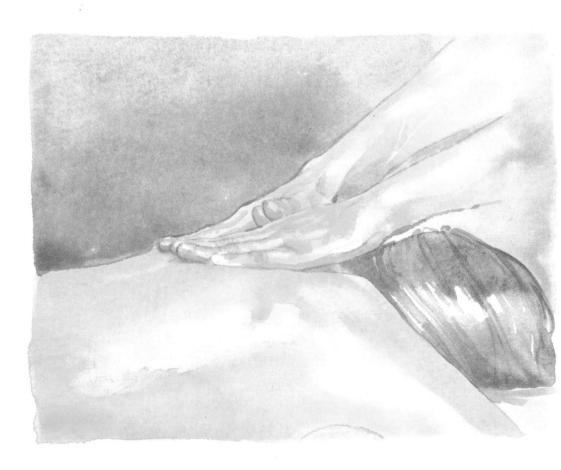

The One Finger Stroke

The One Finger Stroke uses the tip of the middle finger. Place your first finger over the middle finger (see illustration, below) to keep the pressure in the stroke even. This is the most sensitive of all strokes and is used to move energy in a refined way, rather like "teasing" energy along.

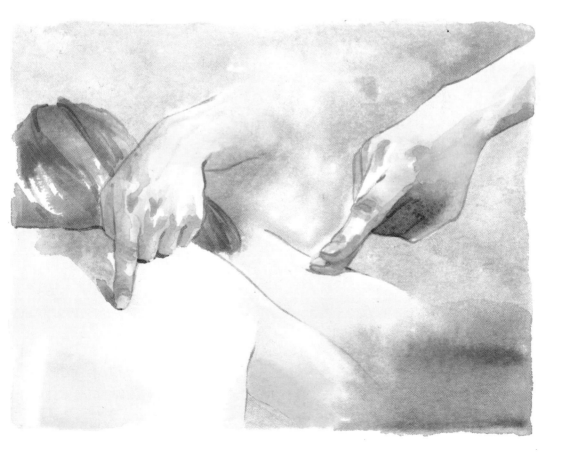

The Pulling Stroke

Use the Pulling Stroke to pull along the side of the body.
Start the stroke with your hand in a soft, clasp-like position,
your thumbs on the upper side, and your palms and
fingertips gently maintaining contact with the underside of
your partner's body (see illustration, below). Apply the
pressure more with the strength of your arms than by
clasping your hands.

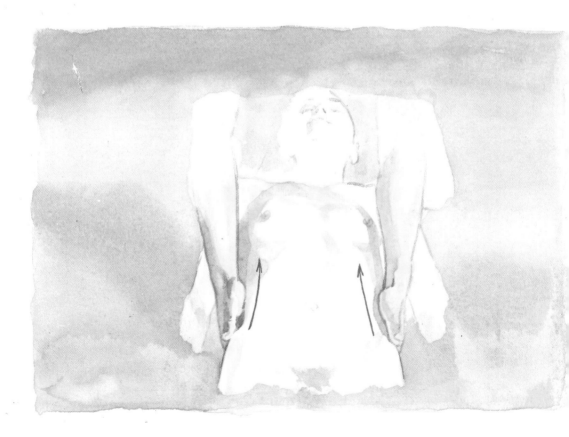

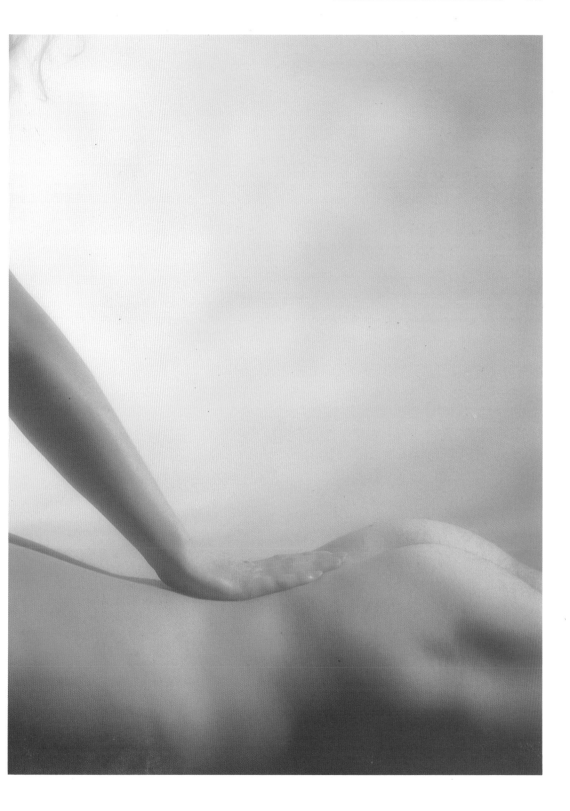

The sequence of the massage

The massage follows a specific sequence. It is divided into three parts: a preparation sequence (see pp. 94-9) opens the energy channels of your body, and prepares them for the main sequence. The main sequence (see pp. 100-85) on the back, then the front of the body, stirs the sexual energy, then guides this energy throughout the body. If followed as described, this main sequence will take you through a wave motion of excitation followed by periods of relaxation (see chart, opposite).

A short sequence that focuses on the face brings the massage to a conclusion. This is designed to settle your partner's body energy at a normal level and prepare your partner to re-enter normal consciousness. If you decide to let the main section of the massage flow on into sexual activity, this final sequence is still a suitable way to finish.

Peaks and valleys

When a wave of sexual energy reaches peak level, we experience the entire orgasm at once, tingling, buzzing, and vibrant with the heat and passion of sexual fire. It is as if each cell of the body is bursting with life force, yearning for release into oneness.

During the valleys of relaxation, the pressure of sexual force subsides gradually, and it is as if the body almost enters everyday reality. The whole body can relax and renew itself.

Energy wave motion chart

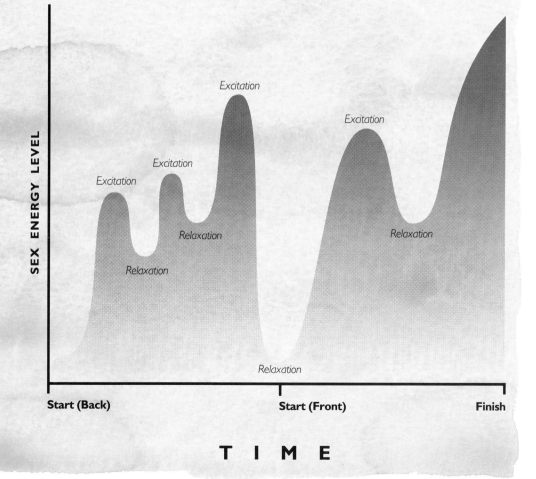

SEX ENERGY LEVEL

Excitation

Excitation

Excitation

Relaxation

Relaxation

Excitation

Relaxation

Relaxation

Start (Back)   **Start (Front)**   **Finish**

T I M E

The spaces between

In contrast to most western massage techniques, where the giver maintains continuous contact with the receiver throughout an entire massage session, Taoist massage emphasizes regular breaks in contact with your partner throughout the session. These intervals are sometimes punctuated by resting positions (see box, below).

While you are changing positions, for example from behind your partner's back to between their legs, you create the space for your partner's body consciousness to assimilate the information so far received, and to prepare to receive more.

Although you are not touching, the energy that surrounds your bodies remains linked. Make use of the spaces in between the touching, just as a musical composer makes use of the spaces between notes, without which music would be a mere wall of sound.

Resting positions

The massage sequence is punctuated by resting positions. Your hand rests, passive, alive, on key energy positions on your partner's body. A natural healing energy is transmitted through the hand. This happens of its own accord, without mental interference (see Wu Wei, p. 38). The healing energy is experienced as a comforting warmth, on a key area such as the sacrum. The resting positions are specifically designed to give time for recentring yourself and your partner. Use them also if at any time during the massage you find that your attention wanders from what you are doing. Throughout the massage sequence, the resting positions, hands-on massage, and the spaces between (see above), produce three distinct, contrasting experiences.

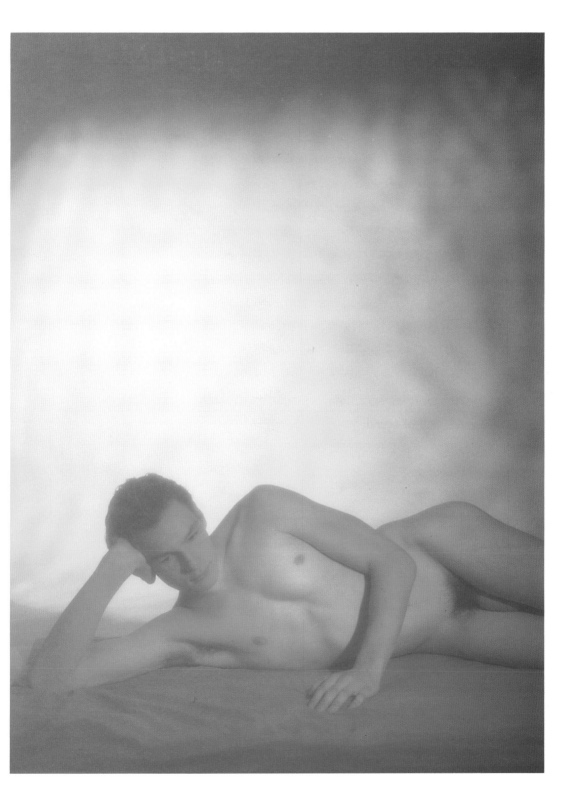

Timing

For each part of the massage sequence, we give an
approximate guideline to how long to continue each
movement. This can only be a guide, which you will refine
for yourself as you perform the massage. Each giver and each
receiver is unique in tastes and receptivity.

Generally allow up to an hour for one massage session,
giver to receiver. You may find that with practice you can
achieve a total healing session within half an hour. It is not
important, as long as the entire sequence is followed with
your mind fully immersed in it, and as long as it is
performed without rushing. Take turns as giver and receiver
if you want to enjoy every moment of both giving and
receiving the massage. When you have become familiar with
the movements of this massage sequence, and if you have
only a short time available, you may want to reduce the
number of techniques and concentrate on a few only. If so,
turn to the bottom of page 186 for a suggestion for selected
techniques that will take very little time to perform.

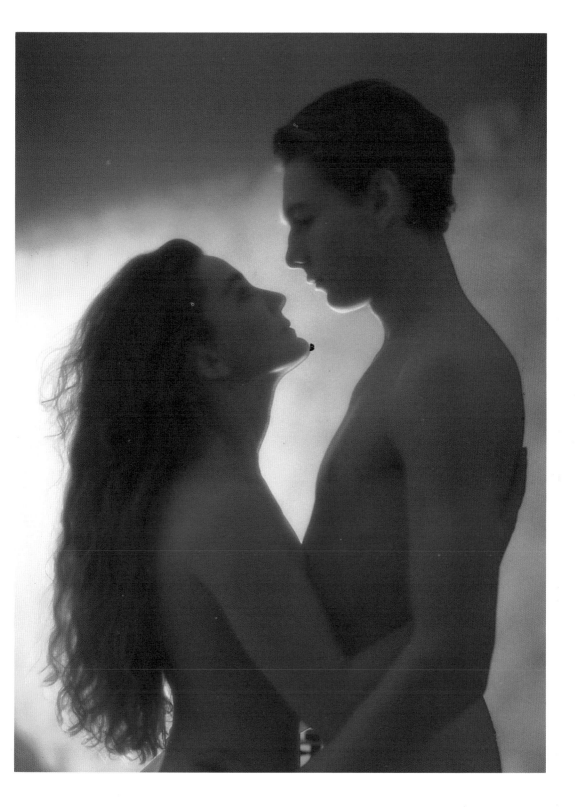

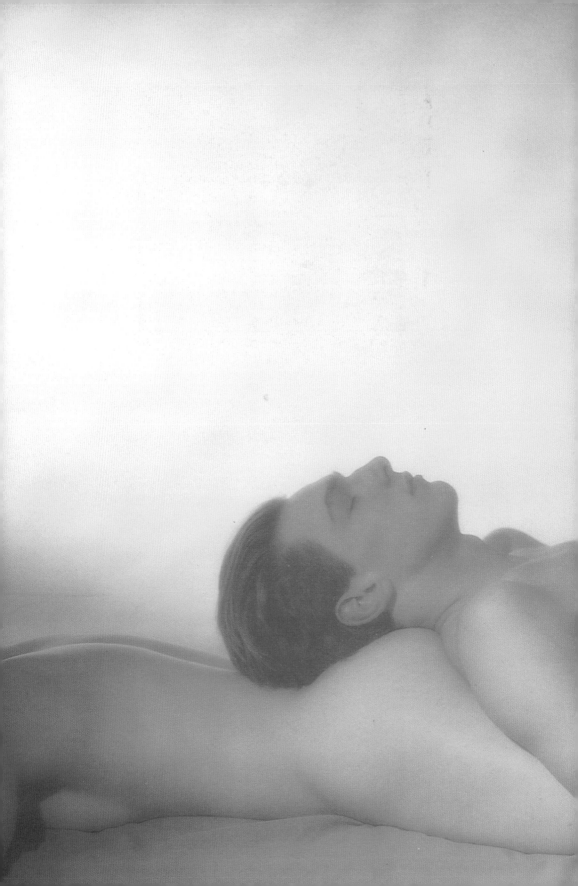

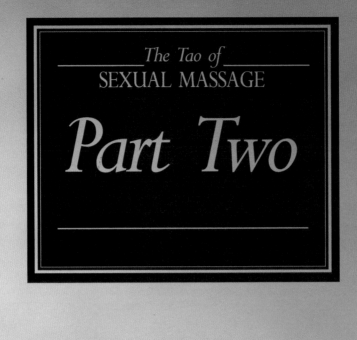

The Tao of
SEXUAL MASSAGE

Part Two

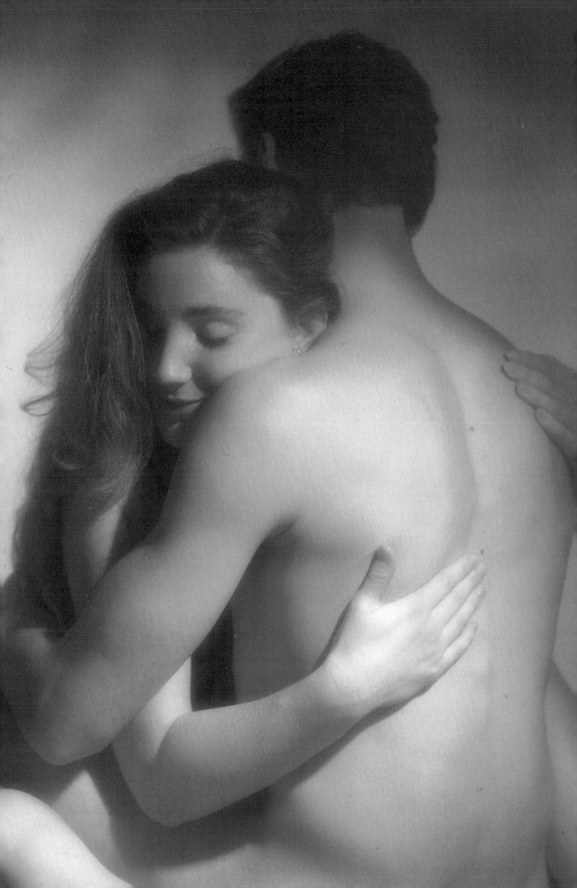

Chapter Five

MANUAL OF TECHNIQUES
BACK SEQUENCE

THE first half of the main sequence works on the back. This is less threatening for the receiver than a massage on the front of the body, and as a result you will gain greater access to your partner's energy field (see p. 26).

You must first clear the obstructions built up by the tensions of daily life, using the series of holds described on pages 94-9. This Preparation Sequence is simple and non-threatening, and yet has an immense effect on the receiver's state of physical relaxation and mental peace. It allows the emotions to settle, the mind to clear, and the body to relax, opening the body's energy field, ready for healing.

Remember to discuss with your partner the way you would like to conduct the session (see p. 65). Remember, too, that you can perform the sequence in any way that you like. You may wish to take turns with your partner. And, once you are familiar with the massage sequence, it might be appropriate to select parts of it (see box, p. 186), and perform those on each other.

The back sequence has a strong and stimulating effect on the body's sexual energy. When you complete it, the receiver will be sufficiently at ease to turn over for the next part of the sequence.

PREPARATION
Pulling the Temples

At the start of a massage session the recipient is usually inclined to be judgemental and resistant. This hold on the sides and the front of the head cuts out judgement, so that your partner feels open and receptive.

Preparing for the massage in this way instantly releases the day's stress. It also helps to ease headaches, eye strain, and blocked sinuses.

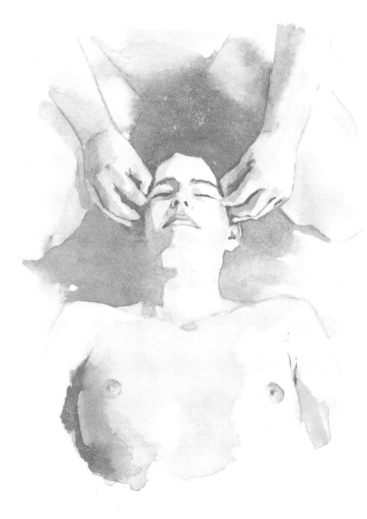

Pulling the Temples
Gently take hold of the soft skin at the indentations of the temples, using your thumbs and forefingers. Slowly pull the skin away from the temples, stretching it across the forehead. Visualize the swirl of spinning thought evaporating from your partner's head. Maintain the hold lightly at the temples for about a minute, while you breathe and relax.

Pulling the Upper Chest

Emotional stress tends to accumulate in the form of tension in the upper chest. This hold will help to release some of this tension, so that your partner can be emotionally more free to enjoy a sensual massage.

By pulling the tissue across this part of the chest you are encouraging fresh blood and energy to stimulate the lungs and thymus gland. This eases your partner's breathing and helps to strengthen the immune system.

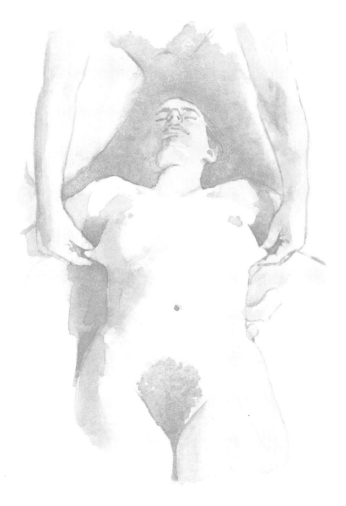

Pulling the Upper Chest

With your fingers and thumbs take hold of the flesh at both sides of the upper chest, next to the armpits. Firmly, but gently, pull the flesh away from the ribs. This creates a stretch across the upper chest. Maintain for about one minute.

As you hold the position, breathe and relax. Visualize emotional hurt and confusions escaping from your partner's chest.

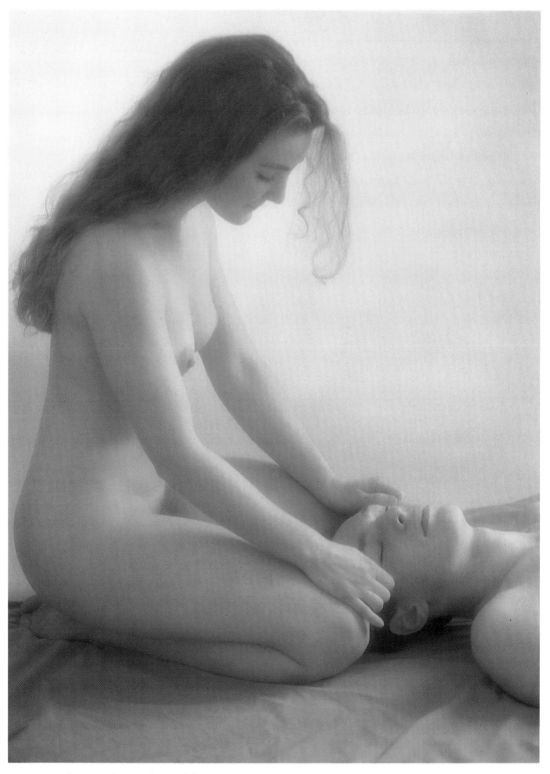

Pulling the Temples (see p. 94)

Pulling the Upper Abdomen

During daily activity the diaphragm - a strong muscle that operates the respiratory mechanism - may become tense. This happens as a normal response to bad news, emotional upset, or any information that is hard to digest. The tension prevents complete exhalation of each breath. For your partner to relax fully, it is imperative for the breathing mechanism to ease.

This technique stimulates the most important stress release point, the solar plexus. The diaphragm will relax immediately; this encourages full and freer breathing.

Solar Plexus

Pulling the Upper Abdomen

With your thumbs and fingers, take hold of the flesh at the sides of the lower ribs, level with the solar plexus, and pull it away from the rib bones.

Maintain this hold for about one minute, stretching the flesh across the upper abdomen.

Visualize your partner in a state of total self acceptance.

Pulling the Lower Abdomen

Stretching the flesh across the lower abdomen allows your partner to feel comfortable about the sexual part of the body, without the giver having to touch it physically. It releases the deep-rooted tension that accumulates in the lower abdomen, which arises from survival fears, repressed sexuality, and irregular intestinal movements.

Visualize your partner's sexual shame and inhibition slowly dispersing, like fog in the sun.

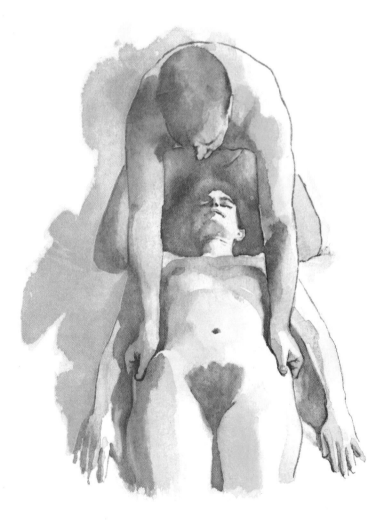

Pulling the Lower Abdomen
Take hold of the flesh at the sides of the hip bones. Pull away from the bone on both sides. Hold for about one minute, stretching the flesh across the lower abdomen.

Pulling the Hips

This stretch releases another major point of tension, the Gate of Mortality, at the perineum (see p. 118). The Gate of Mortality tenses as we struggle to define and redefine our identity, and as we meet the stimulus of our daily information input. It is essential to release tension at this point in order to allow a healthy flow of blood and energy in the genital area. When this point is relaxed and "open", you are at one with your entire personal consciousness.

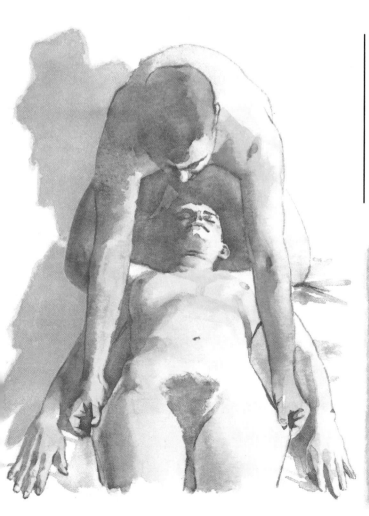

Pulling the Hips

Take hold of the flesh at the top of the outer thighs. Hold it between thumbs and fingers and pull away from the joint at the top of the thigh (see p. 82).

Maintain the hold, subtly stretching the flesh across the lower pubic region for about one minute.

As you hold the position, visualize the Gate of Mortality opening, and think of your partner being in a state of peace, knowing his or her true identity.

The Meeting of
One Hundred Energies
The Gate of Mortality is the
opposite of the Meeting of One
Hundred Energies point at the
crown of the head. When this point
is open, you are at one with the
consciousness of the entire universe.

BACK SEQUENCE

Having completed the preparation techniques (pp. 94-9), your partner's emergy field is now open and ready for the massage sequence. Ask your partner to turn over slowly and lie face down.

Resting Position - Hand Between Shoulder Blades

By resting a healing hand between the shoulder blades, you will, with repetition, help your partner to become free of the negative emotional stockpile that develops in this area (see box, facing page). Your partner will noticeably relax more deeply; this allows the trust level between you to rise, ready for the subsequent techniques.

The Crimson Palace

The area of the body between the shoulder blades is like the "back yard" of the heart centre (see pp. 132-3). Known as the Rear Door of the Crimson Palace, it is one of the most important tension release points in the entire body.

This is where we tend to throw our emotional garbage - those issues that we cannot immediately resolve. Eventually this garbage heap starts to affect the heart centre, in the front of the chest - also known as the Crimson Palace. It becomes home to unresolved and painful emotional issues. This in turn can lead to chronic tension of the muscles in the area, which will in time cause postural distortions of the spine. It will also eventually affect the heart and lungs.

Strength is needed to hold this unnecessary tension. This strength comes from the kidney region of the lower back, which having been issued, will leave the kidneys weak or under-energized, thus weakening the lower back. At the same time the tension inhibits blood, nerve, and energy flow to the brain and, with the head thrown forward by the curve of the spine, thoughts will tend to become cloudy and grim. Attitude to life and everyday situations will become unbalanced.

Generating energy from your palm

Visualize a great furnace, burning in the palm of your right hand. Now gently place your palm between the shoulder blades of your partner's back, fingers pointing toward the head. Slowly apply a small amount of pressure, bringing the mid-point of your palm in contact with the back.

Feel as if you are lengthening your partner's spine and broadening the back. Let the warmth of your hand flow through your palm; picture a comforting force permeating the back, out to the sides, and deep down into the chest. Maintain this position for about half a minute.

When you have finished, draw your hand away slowly, as if pulling silk from a cocoon.

Jiggling the Column

Jiggling the Column works in the opposite direction from the flow of energy moving up from the sacrum (see box, facing page). It temporarily breaks up postural tensions and confuses the part of the mind that has invested energy in keeping them fixed. It then becomes possible to create a more suitable physical context for a correct energy flow.

Clearing the column of these energy moulds and obstructions also has a positive effect on sexual patterns. The technique helps to break up expectations of sexual gratification, leaving your partner's mind open to experience something new.

Jiggling the Column

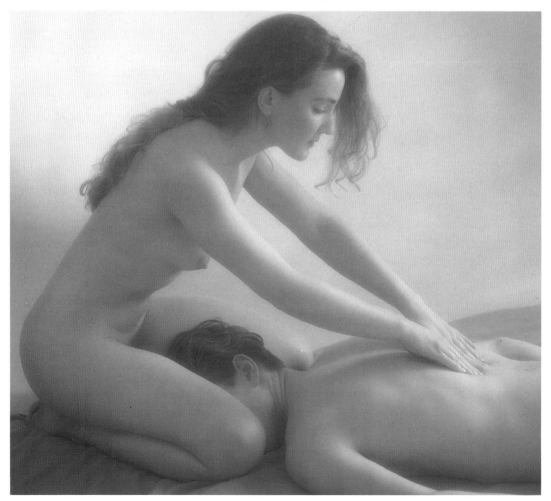

Jiggling the Column

Place the finger pads of both hands at the base of the 7th cervical vertebra, the large protruding neck bone. Imagine that you are kneading dough with a rolling pin, back and forth, quickly. Now make this rolling motion with your finger pads on the vertebra in front of them. Roll the skin back and forth quickly, firmly, and lightly. Your partner's body will begin to rock back and forth a little.

After establishing the rhythm, let your hands automatically start to move down the spine using your partner's rocking motion. Work toward the sacrum, rocking back and forth over the vertebrae. Allow this downward movement to last about 30 seconds.

When you have "jiggled" the column to the sacrum, begin again from the top. Repeat twice.

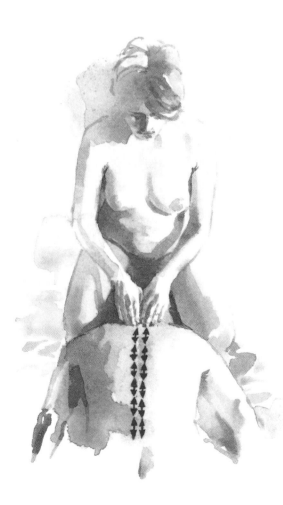

The Channel of Control

The spinal column is like a flag pole, held vertical by the muscles surrounding the spine. It houses the Channel of Control, through which your sexual energies travel upward from the sacrum to the brain.

This energy controls human existence and subsequently the functioning of the entire organism. The central focus of Taoist medicine is to clear its often obstructed path up the column to the brain to produce a state of enlightenment and perfect health. This work is always necessary because, in most cases, negative thought patterns that have built up over time cause negative postural holding patterns. These make the muscles of the spinal column compress, and in turn impair the passageway of energy through the spinal column.

Resting Position - Sacrum

This resting position is one of the most powerful universal healing holds. It immediately makes your partner feel safe and whole at a fundamental level, like a baby, secure in its mother's arms. While you hold the position, you may notice your partner falling into a semi-dream state, which indicates an effective altering of consciousness.

This resting position can also assist with deep-seated sexual trauma, sciatic nerve pain, weakness of the legs, lower back pain, and problems of the prostate gland and uterus.

Resting your palm

Envisage a red-hot flame, burning in the palm of your right hand. Place your palm softly on the sacrum, fingers pointing up the spine. Imagine the heat spreading out through your hand into your partner's sacrum and from there in all directions, even permeating the genitals with its healing, nurturing warmth. Press down gently, to broaden your partner's hips with your palm, while lengthening the lower spine with your fingers. Maintain this hold for about one minute, then lift your hand slowly.

The Gate of the Spine

The sacrum is known as the Gate of the Spine. It is the rear store-house of the body's sexual energy and vitality. "Sacrum" is a Latin word meaning sacred place. To unlock the powerful energies of this sacred place and allow them to circulate around the body via the spine, it is often only necessary to lay on a warm, healing hand.

Once the sacral area is relaxed, the gate opens and energy can flow into the Channel of Control (see p. 103) and rise upward.

Opening the Gate of the Spine

This massage enhances the work of the previous technique. As before, it assists with deep-seated sexual trauma, sciatic nerve pain, weakness of the legs, lower back pain, prostate gland and uterine problems, as well as urinary problems, impotence, and vaginismus (see p. 187) - vaginal spasms that make sexual intercourse impossible.

Opening the Gate

Place your hands on each side of the sacrum, fingers toward the head. Then with the pads of your thumbs, push up the mid-line of the sacrum with alternating strokes about two inches (5cm) long, first with the left thumb, and then with the right. A right and a left stroke takes about three seconds. Maintain this stroking action with even speed and light pressure, for one minute. The lighter your strokes, the stronger the effect.

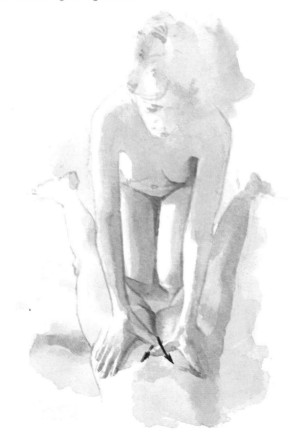

Visualizing the energy

Visualize sending the fiery energy held in the sacrum up the spine, like billiard balls from a cue. Each stroke sends a volley of energy balls up the Channel of Control and into the brain.

Feeling the energy

As the energy climbs the spine, your partner may experience a feeling of euphoria. At the same time, energy is magnifying in front of the sacrum and throughout the genital region. This energy release may induce sexual arousal, especially if you employ sensitivity and a light touch with your thumbs.

Climbing the Column

Having awakened the powerful force in the sacrum and cleared its path (see pp. 104-5), you can assist its continuing climb up the spine through the Channel of Control.

This massage will release the spine and its surrounding muscles. It may also relieve stiffness and pain in the lower, middle, and upper back.

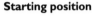

Starting position

Place your left hand on the sacrum, fingers pointing forward. Wait until your palm has "settled" into the sacrum. Do not use undue pressure. Now place your right palm just in front of your left, along the spine, fingers pointing to the head.

Visualizing the energy

Visualize lengthening and smoothing the spine like a block of clay into a long, straight line. Each stroke sends waves of energy upward to the brain.

As you move your hand, imagine clearing away your partner's debris of residual tension, accumulated over a lifetime.

While your left palm maintains and stimulates sexual energy, your right palm helps to disperse the resulting fire, warming your partner's heart and mind.

Feeling the energy

Your partner may experience a surge of strength from the enhanced flow, filling and empowering the entire organism and enlivening the genital region.

Completing the technique

Slowly and deliberately, with light pressure at first, push your right palm up along the spine, vertebra by vertebra, using the Flat Hand Stroke (see p. 80), until your finger pads are pressing into the base of the skull. Maintain an even speed for this movement. This stroke should take about twenty seconds. Lift your hand gently and repeat the movement for approximately three minutes, increasing the pressure with each ascending stroke, but keeping the pressure of the left hand steady.

Vitality and energy
The Channel of Control leads the sexual energy up the spine (see p. 103), and disperses the energy to all the organs lying along its path. The organs assimilate this pure energy. Your partner will feel more vital and energized. When added to the stimulation of sexual energy in the sacrum, this will lead to great feelings of enthusiasm and desire for sexual contact.

Supporting the Column Part I

After lengthening the spine in Climbing the Column (see pp. 106-7), this technique releases excess tension in the supporting muscles, and allows the spine to "float upward", elongating it further. The resulting lightness felt in the entire body lightens the overall mood and renders your partner playful like a child. The movement can relieve muscular tension all over the back; it also enhances overall balance and integrity. Sexual energy and desire will increase in the genital region, though this may not yet be evident.

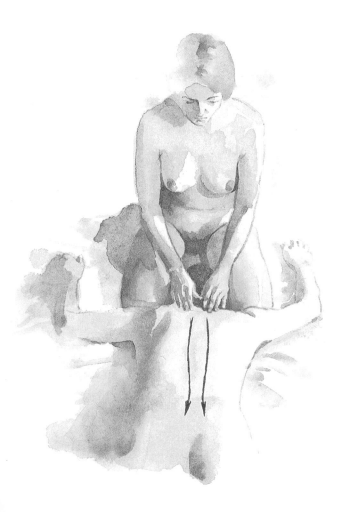

Starting the movement

Place your palms either side of the spine, fingers pointing toward the sacrum. Keep your back straight and shoulders fully relaxed.

Using your body weight (not the strength of your arms) push both hands firmly and steadily downward toward the sacrum using the Flat Hand Stroke (see p. 80).

The Bladder Channel

Running down each side of the spine lies the Bladder Channel. This transports fluid kidney energy to all the organs in turn as it passes along the length of the back. For example, between the shoulder blades lie entry points to the Heart Channel. Next in line lie entry points to the channels of the liver, spleen, kidney, intestines, bladder, and sexual organs. As you pass your hands down along the length of the Bladder Channel toward the sacrum, its invigorating Water energy will bathe each of the organs in turn. This helps to keep each organ lubricated and healthy. It also takes excess mental energy from the upper body downward to the sexual region for regeneration and reuse as sexual fire.

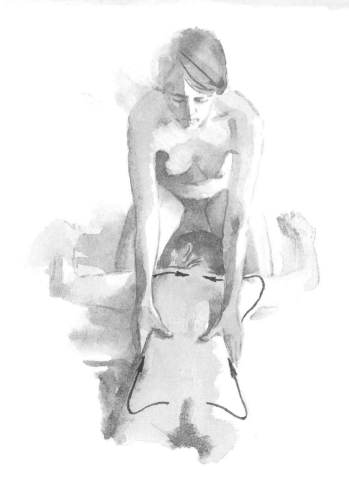

Completing the technique

At the sacrum, separate your hands to the sides, one to each hip, and then pull upward along the sides of the torso to the armpits (see p. 82). As you move upward, let your fingers pull up the sides and over the front of the ribs, while your thumb pads pull up over your partner's back.

When you reach the armpits, circle your hands around the outsides of the shoulder blades, until the fingers of both hands are once again at the starting position, ready for the next cycle. This comprises one cycle, lasting about 25 seconds. Repeat the movement for about three minutes.

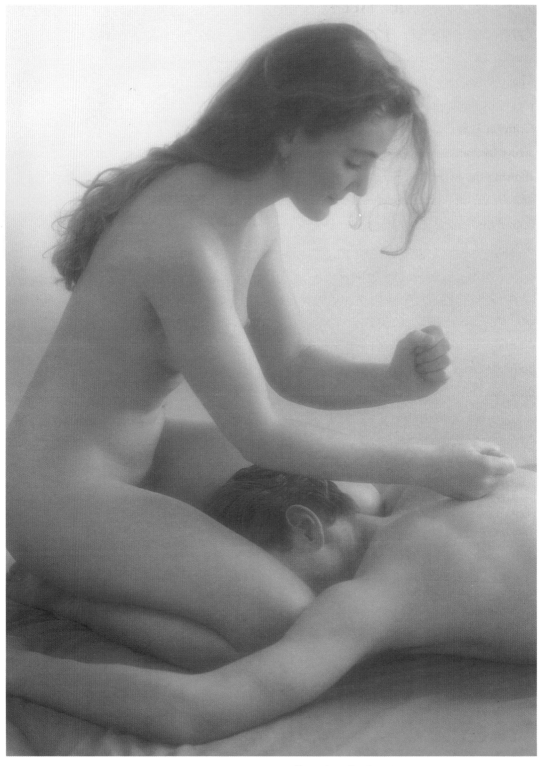

Pounding the Rear Door of the Crimson Palace

Pounding the Rear Door of the Crimson Palace

This percussion technique (see p. 78) works on the "hump" region of the upper back, behind the heart centre, or Crimson Palace (see p. 101). It clears the effects of pride and arrogance, and releases tension from the lung region, allowing the heart energy to flow more freely. As a result it lifts the mood and makes your partner feel happy and optimistic. People often laugh spontaneously during this technique - a sure sign that they are releasing tension.

This release of tension from the heart and lung region helps such conditions as tachycardia, angina, palpitations, asthma, emphysema, anxiety, insomnia, and certain manic disorders. It is also an effective method for achieving sudden body awareness in a person who is completely immersed in their own mental energy.

Feeling the energy

A moment or two after you have stopped pounding, your partner will experience a sensation as if energy were fizzing in the upper back. This is the release of the Joyous Fire of the Heart.

Pounding the Rear Door
Make a relaxed, fairly loose fist with each hand (see p. 78). Position your fists in the air above the region between the shoulder blades. With a slow, steady, even tempo let the weight of your relaxed fists fall one at a time on to your partner's back, alternating strokes as if making a slow drum roll. Feel as if each beat is penetrating into your partner's chest. Be sure to keep your shoulders, elbows, and wrists flexible and relaxed. Enjoy the process. Keep your breathing slow and steady.

Continue the percussion for about one minute, then slowly come to a natural stop.

Pounding the Gate of the Spine

Having stimulated the heart energy (see p. 111) it is now time to stir the Original Fire at the Gate of the Spine - the sexual energy stored in the sacrum. This will cause the two energies to mingle in the sacral region, producing the true sexual urge.

The technique has proved to be particularly helpful in treating weakness of the lower limbs caused by multiple sclerosis. It is also helpful as a treatment for poor circulation in the legs, numbness of the lower limbs, impotence, vaginismus (see p. 187), urinary and bladder problems, and weakness of the lower back.

Caution

Do not use this technique if you suffer from spinal injury, or if you are undergoing serious chiropractic or osteopathic treatment.

Pounding the Gate

Begin this routine with your shoulders fully relaxed and open. Visualize enough space under each of your armpits to fit a golden apple. Imagine your elbow joints are expanded and floating on a cushion of air. Let your forearms feel empty, and keep your wrists loose.

Make a soft fist shape with your hands (see p. 78). Place your fists on the sacrum, and with the bouncing energy of a monkey, start to play a light, slow drum roll of even strokes and tempo.

As you breathe and relax, let the tempo of the drum roll automatically accelerate, maintaining an even and light pressure.

Continue this percussion for close to one minute, then decelerate gradually, until your fists eventually come to rest with one final stroke on the sacrum. Let your fists rest there lightly while you check your breath and allow your energy to settle.

Drumming the fire

The pelvic region is the storehouse of the sexual energy of the kidneys. Drumming on the sacrum vibrates this fire, intensifies it, and keeps it active.

Remember to keep your arms, shoulders, and wrists relaxed and feeling "rubbery", otherwise you will transmit your own tension through your fists into this extremely sensitive and receptive area of your partner's body.

Feeling the energy

Your partner will feel a strong fizzing sensation moving from the sacrum to the genitals and up along the spinal column to the Cave of Original Spirit in the midbrain. This fizzing is the Original Fire of Life, the catalyst for sexual force in the genitals and for generative force in the brain. Your partner will probably feel a warm glow throughout the whole body and a sudden increase in desire.

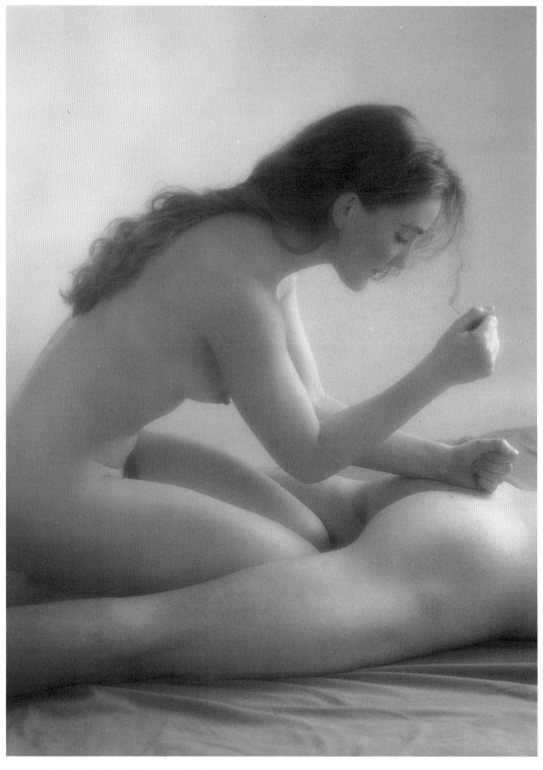

Pounding the Gate of the Spine (see pp. 112-3)

Mixing the Original and Joyous Fires

You can now complete the process of the previous two techniques by blending the Joyous Fire of the heart with the Original Fire of the sacrum. This produces the true sexual urge in the genitals and, by stirring it, takes it to a stronger level. The effects of the technique are similar to those of detonating an explosive in a confined space. It generates enormous heat, which rushes into the genitals and produces a strong sexual reaction.

This technique strengthens the kidneys, augmenting strength and resistance to disease. This in itself produces a remarkable increase in sexual energy and desire.

Starting the movement
Place one palm on each shoulder blade, fingers pointing toward the sacrum, along the bilateral Bladder Channel (see p. 109). Keep your back straight and, breathing slowly and regularly, push slowly but firmly using the Flat Hand Stroke (see p. 80) along the pathway on each side of the spine to the sacrum. Then pull back upward along the spine itself, using your thumbs instead of your palms.

Benefits for the giver
This technique, if performed in the correct way, can be a good exercise for the masseur, strengthening the upper body, and the cardiovascular and respiratory systems.

(Mixing the Original and Joyous Fires contd.)

Completing the technique

Begin to accelerate the movement gradually with each stroke. As your movement speeds up, you will naturally begin to reduce the massage area to the part of the back between the lower ribs and the sacrum.

After about one minute, or as soon as you are aware of a heat build-up on your partner's back, stop suddenly, palms resting over the lumbar region of the back (see above). Gently rock your partner toward and away from you. Let the heat from your palms permeate the kidney region and penetrate deeply through to the abdomen. This gentle rocking motion will physically stimulate the outer genitals.

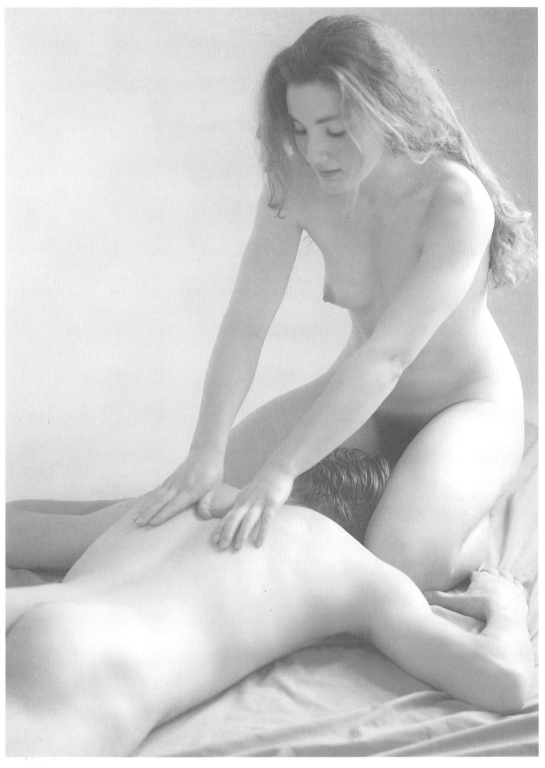

Mixing the Original and Joyous Fires (see p. 115)

Supporting the Column Part II

After stirring the spinal forces to boiling point, it is now time to spread them around the body at the new intensified level, especially to the genital region. By now your partner should have moved observably into a wonderfully pleasurable state of consciousness. This part of the massage sequence releases all remaining back tension. The technique is especially helpful in alleviating sexual guilt, shame, and tensions held in the region of the anus that are the result of fear and anxiety.

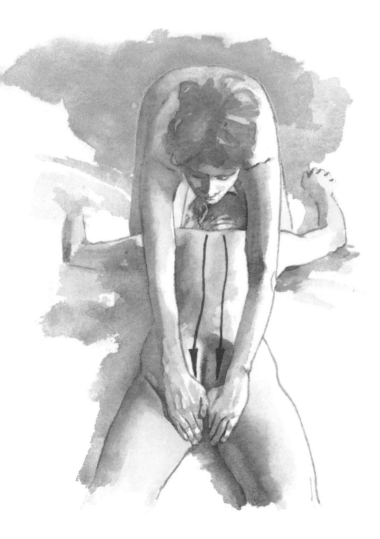

Starting the movement

Place your palms on each side of the top of the spine, fingers pointing toward the sacrum. Using the Flat Hand Stroke (see p. 80), push both hands slowly down toward the sacrum. Then continue down over the buttocks. Let your thumbs lightly brush along the "valley floor" between the buttocks, and just past the anus to the perineum (see also p. 163).

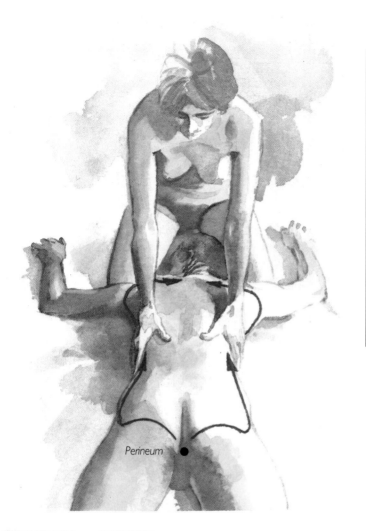

Perineum

Completing the technique

Push your fingers forward to the backs of the thighs, then separate your hands, one to each outer thigh, and pull up your partner's sides to the armpits (see p. 82). Turn your hands over the shoulders and let them meet again at the top of the spine to complete the movement.

Start with a light pressure, almost tickling your partner, then gradually increase pressure from cycle to cycle to a firm but comfortable level. Then begin to lighten the pressure, and end with a lightly pressured cycle. Only use a light pressure over the anal region and perineum.

Allow yourself up to 30 seconds to complete each cycle. Continue this sequence for up to five minutes.

Visualizing the energy

These strokes link the energies of the rear torso and the backs of the thighs. Kidney energy, which controls sexuality, is stored in the torso, and the backs of the thighs store much of the body's withheld sexual energy.

Feeling the energy

Throughout this technique your partner will experience an intensified sexual energy, which may well be clear to observe. Most people just cannot resist moving their hips, in a delighted response to this manipulation.

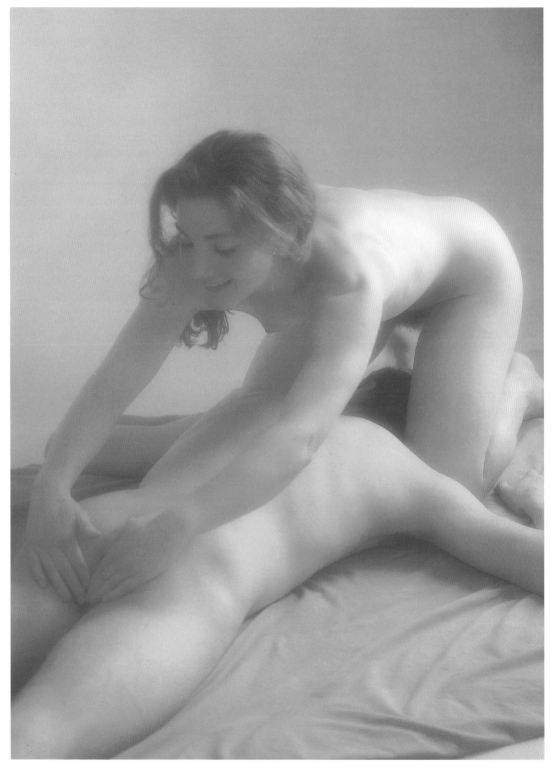

Supporting the Column Part II (see pp. 118-9)

Resting Position – Top of Thighs

This hold signals a short rest for your partner and for you. During this time your partner's body and mind will assimilate the stimulation received in the massage sequence so far.

The sexual energy level (see pp. 84-5) will plateau at slightly below peak during this exercise, after which your partner will be ready for the next series of techniques.

Magnetic power from your hands

Visualize a furnace burning in the palm of your hand. Place your palm across the backs of both legs, just below the base of the buttocks. Imagine that the furnace in your hand has a great magnetic pulling power, attracting your partner's sexual energy.

Rock your partner gently from side to side for about 30 seconds, then gradually release.

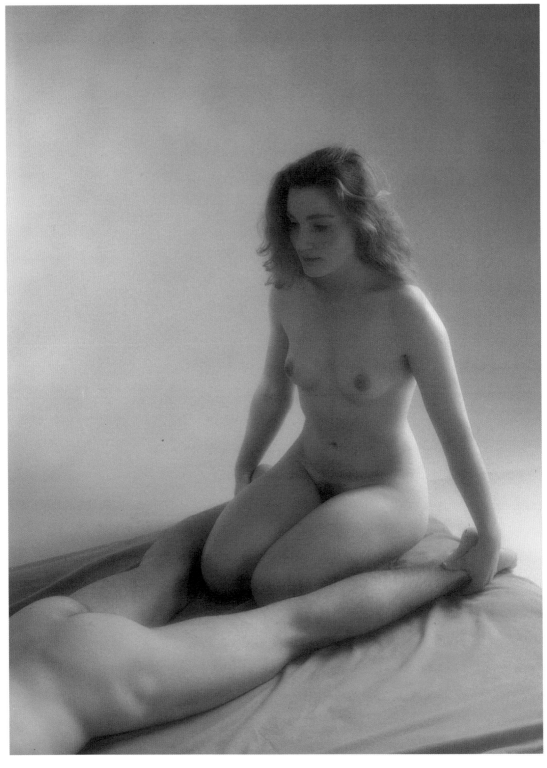

Resting Position - Outer Ankle

Resting Position - Outer Ankle

This hold provides a stationary resting point from which you can gain strength to continue with the massage.

By holding both ankles in this way you are contacting important points on the Bladder Channel (see pp. 28-9). Mild stimulation of this channel helps to increase overall body strength and outer layer protection. It also invigorates the two sides of the brain and the eyes.

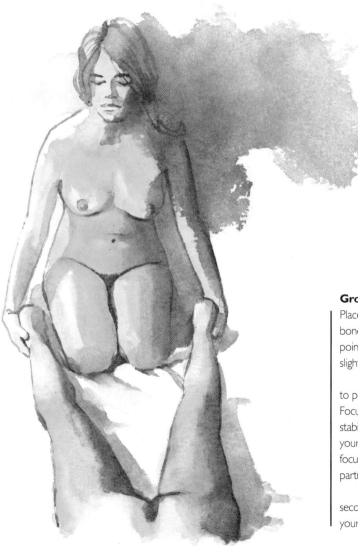

Grounding the energies

Place one palm over each outer ankle bone. Turn your partner's feet to point the toes inward, and the heels slightly outward.

Allow the warmth of your palms to permeate the entire ankle region. Focus your mind on maintaining, stabilizing, and most important, leading your partner's energy and mental focus downward. This "grounds" your partner's energy.

Maintain this hold for about 30 seconds, to let your energy levels and your breathing settle.

Leading the Water

This technique frees your partner of sexual inhibitions. By working on the backs of the legs, you can release your partner's inclination to resist new experiences, both in the emotional and sexual realms.

Do not rush this massage. It is a highly sensual technique and the effects of sexual excitation may be clearly visible. For men who suffer from premature ejaculation this massage is recommended on a regular basis.

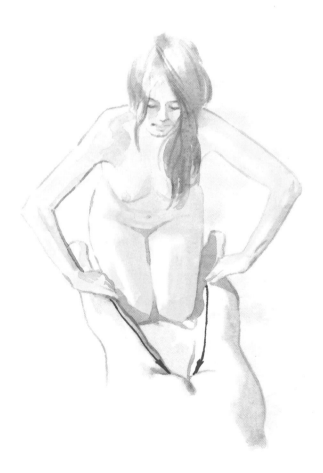

Starting the movement
From the resting position (see p. 123), move your palms to the inner ankle bones, then lightly stroke up the insides of the calves, knees, and backs of the thighs.

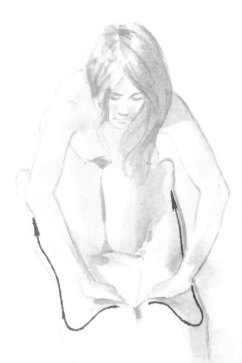

Completing the technique

When your hands reach the perineum (see left), separate them, one over each buttock, to the hips, and pull down (see p. 82) the outer backs and sides of the legs, ending at the outer ankles. On your downward stroke, trace your thumbs along the median line of each leg (see below).

This comprises one cycle of the movement. Each cycle can last to up to 30 seconds.

Your partner will probably find this very stimulating sexually and will move the hips in response.

Yin and Yang channels in the leg

On the upward stroke of this movement, the giver is stimulating the three Yin leg energy channels of the kidney, liver, and spleen. The downward movement in turn stimulates the three Yang leg energy channels - the bladder, gall bladder, and stomach. This attunes inner with outer strength and encourages the distribution of fluids.

Pressure and speed

The longer you take on each upward movement and the lighter your touch, the stronger the effect is likely to be. For some people however, a slow, light, touch can be such a strong energetic stimulus that it becomes unbearable. It is best therefore, as in all healing, to follow your intuition and judgement as to the right speed and pressure for this massage.

Stirring the Water

By exciting the powerful meridians in the mid-line of the body, around the buttocks, you are stirring and arousing the "Waters of Sexual Vitality", which provide a basis for the sexual fire. This enables your partner to feel fluid, warm, and soft, while at the same time feeling highly aroused sexually. It is quite normal for female recipients to experience mild orgasms during this procedure.

Stirring the Water
This movement begins at the inner ankle, just like the buttock massage in "Leading the Water" (see pp. 124-5). This time however, when your hands come to the buttocks, let your fingertips brush from the perineum up to the anus. Then part your hands and massage around and over each buttock, then to the sides, spreading the buttocks apart.

Continue by pulling down and turning your hands just under the buttocks, then moving your fingertips across again to the perineum. This comprises one cycle, lasting for about 30 seconds.

Keep in mind that the slower and lighter your strokes, the greater the response you are likely to bring about. Continue this massage by circling over and around the buttocks for about three minutes.

Mid-line meridians
This sequence stimulates three major channels of energy: the Channel of Control, running up the spine to the brain, the Channel of True Function, running up the mid-line of the front of the body, and the Bladder Channel, running from the brain to the heels.

Opening or Closing the Gate of Mortality

The name of this technique describes the choice that you can make to break the sequence of the massage at this point and make love, or to continue the massage. Every time you follow your sexual desire enough to act it out, you are reaffirming your existence on the material plane, and so reaffirming your own mortality. If on the other hand, you transmute the energy behind the desire, you can send the transmuted energy back through the Gate of Mortality, up to the brain, which leads to spiritual immortality and enhanced overall health.

Opening or Closing the Gate of Mortality

From the end of the last cycle of Stirring the Water (see facing page), with your hands resting on the lower part of the buttocks, hold the buttocks apart with your fingers and palms. Now with your right thumb start circling firmly on the perineum. Circle counter-clockwise to maintain the sexual energy at a plateau. Circle clockwise if you want to intensify desire and make love.

Whichever way you choose to circle, continue to do so for about one minute.

Making an agreement
If you have not made an agreement on how to proceed at this point, it is essential to ask your partner now. (See Making an agreement, p. 65).

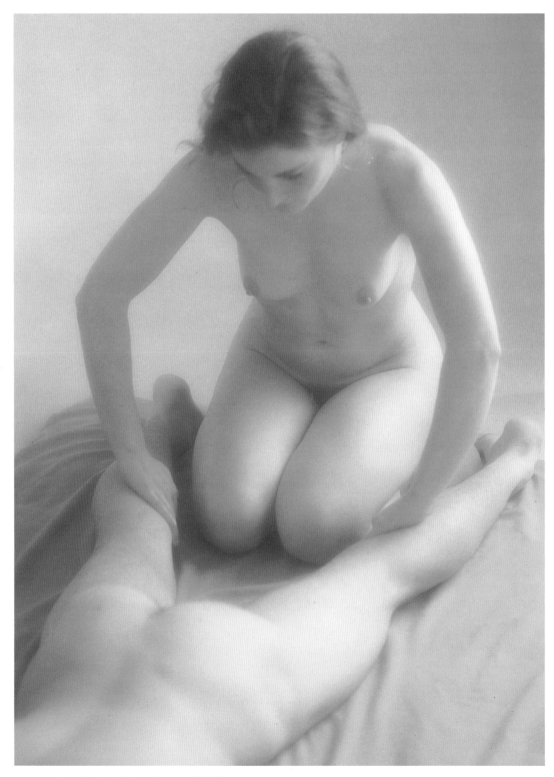

Leading the Water (see pp. 124-5)

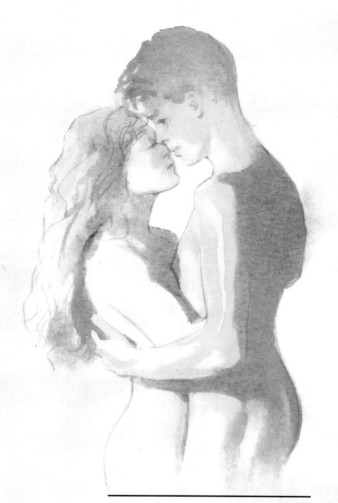

Having completed the massage thus far, sexual energy has been guided through valleys, plateaus, and peaks. It has been made ready for further transmutation into higher energy, using the techniques on pages 94-127, or to increase your sexual enjoyment. If you choose to engage in sexual activity, follow it with the harmonizing and balancing techniques that follow on pages 173-84.

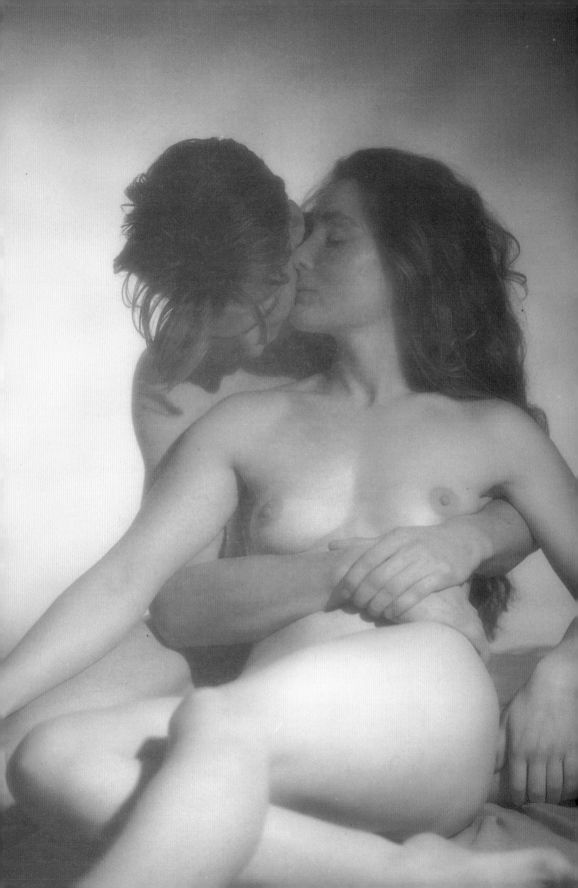

Chapter Six

MANUAL OF TECHNIQUES
FRONT SEQUENCE

THE second half of the main sequence focuses on the front of the body. It begins with a gentle introduction, by performing some simple resting positions. These help you to gain access to your partner's energy field. The massage continues by building up your partner's sexual energy, and moving it through the peaks and valleys of excitation.

The Front Sequence is more stimulating for giver and receiver and, because of the face to face contact, it enables a much closer interplay between both personalities. The Back Sequence of the massage will have prepared you both for the increased level of stimulation.

At the end of the Front Sequence, a short, final series of techniques on the face (see pp. 173-84) balances and harmonizes your partner's feelings. This Final Sequence is designed to help both you and your partner re-enter the normal state of consciousness. You should also use these techniques as a way of ending your session if you have broken the massage sequence at any point to make love.

FRONT SEQUENCE
Resting Position - Heart Centre

The middle of the sternum, or breastbone, is the heart centre, or Crimson Palace (see p. 101). It is the home of the Emperor of the body and an important psychic centre of consciousness. When it is contracted and closed, passion for life is stifled, the mind becomes stagnant and introverted, and the ability to give and receive love is severely impaired.

This position engenders trust and gives you direct access to your partner's energy field. You may see and feel your partner's breathing slow down, as the chest drops and relaxes.

It is essential to open this centre so that your partner feels safe and receptive to the massage that follows.

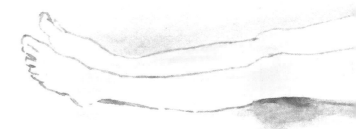

Resting position

Place your left palm along the vertical mid-line of your partner's breastbone, your fingertips on the lower tip of the sternum. Use only light pressure, as if resting your hand on virgin snow, melting it with your body heat.

Feel your palm and finger pads spreading out the breastbone as if to broaden it. Mentally and physically, direct pressure toward your partner's pubic bone without making any actual movement of the hand.

Allow the warmth of your body to flow through your hand into your partner's chest. Your intention is to comfort and heal. Maintain this for about 30 seconds.

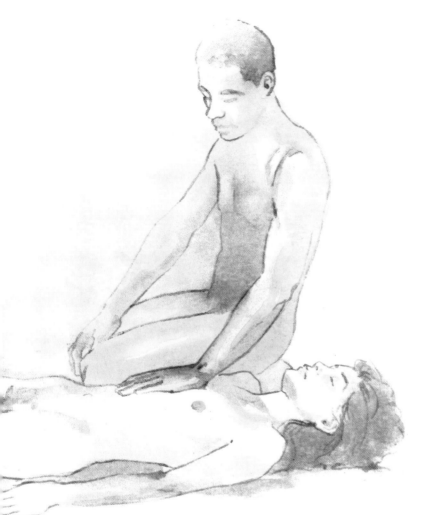

Subtle movements

Although this appears to be a simple position to hold, it is a highly sophisticated technique, involving subtle movement of the small muscles of the arm and hand. It requires sensitivity - an ability to "listen" through your palm. The effects are far-reaching.

Breaking the Flow

Having gained access to your partner's front energy field, and created a sense of security, it is time to break the habitual patterns of the energy flow over the front of the body.

Most of the body's energy channels run up and down the length of the body (see pp. 28-9), and this horizontal massage temporarily breaks the energy flow, in order to introduce a new and healthier passage of energy.

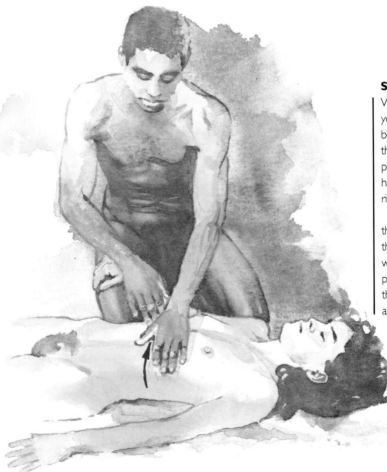

Starting the movement

Visualize a horizontal band across your partner's body, half way between the line of the nipples and the line of the navel. Sitting on your partner's right side, place your left hand at the far side, over the lower ribs on your partner's left side.

Now pull your hand slowly across the band toward you, to the ribs on the right side. Follow this immediately with the right palm, then alternately pulling with left and right palms, across the body. Keep your pressure light and your movements fairly slow.

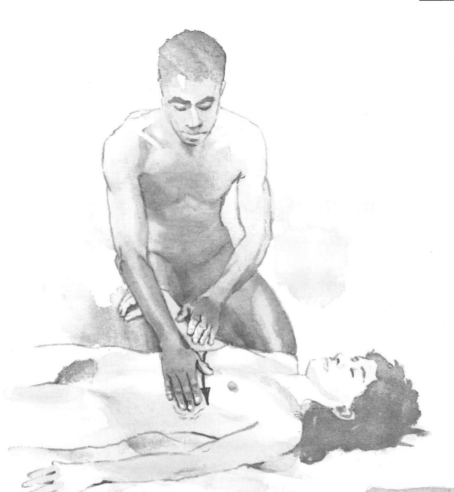

Completing the technique

Repeat these alternate strokes for about half a minute, feeling the upper abdomen grow warm. Then gradually slow down your strokes and let your right palm rest over the lower ribs on the right side for a moment.

Now reverse the movement, pushing your hands across the body, with alternate strokes, from the right side to the left. After 30 seconds or so, slow down and rest your left palm for a moment over the lower ribs on the far side.

Balancing and relaxing

This massage balances the digestive and blood-producing functions of the spleen on the left (see p. 161), with the blood-purifying and releasing energies of the liver on the right. This in turn increases the raw animal vigour of the body, settles the digestive organs, and relaxes the diaphragm, so that breathing can slow down and become deeper.

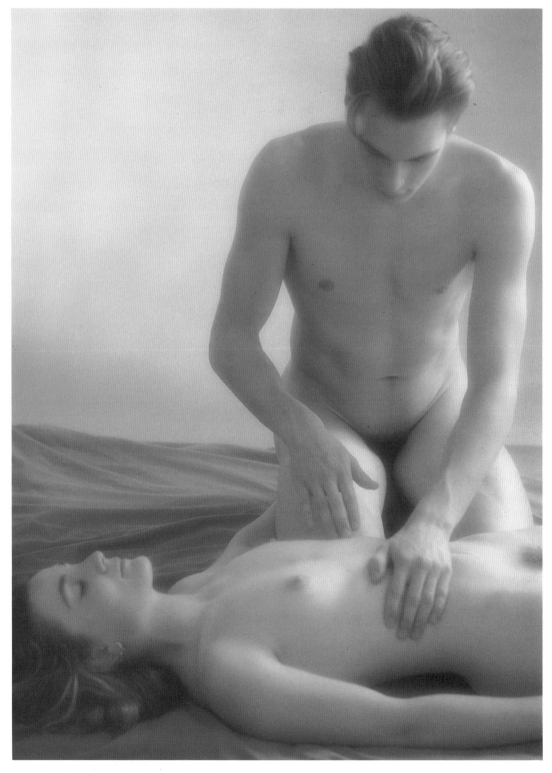

Breaking the Flow (see pp. 134–5)

Resting Position - Solar Plexus

This technique aims to energize the solar plexus; this will tone the entire nervous system and relax the diaphragm. Your partner's breathing will be deeper and more relaxed.

Lack of self acceptance or the presence of any inner conflict immediately translates into tension in the upper abdomen. As this tension is released, levels of self acceptance may rise and inner conflict tends to settle. This change is essential in order for your partner to accept the stimulation of sexual energies that follow in the massage sequence.

Resting on the solar plexus

Rest your left palm on the upper abdomen, below the breastbone, fingers pointing toward the pubic bone. Using only light pressure, direct your hand toward the pubic bone, without moving it. Visualize your palm spreading out the upper abdomen.

Maintain this for about 30 seconds and observe how your partner's breathing slows down and continues to deepen.

The solar plexus

Physiologically, the solar plexus area is the part of the body that accepts and assimilates food. Psychically, the area is responsible for the acceptance and assimilation of new information about the external and internal world.

Building the Fire under the Stove

This circling massage builds up your partner's energy in the lower abdomen, an area known as the Sea of Vitality - the home of the generative force.

If this force is led downward, it manifests as sexual desire and the need for subsequent fulfilment. When this force is led upward, it manifests as overall vitality.

The massage can help ease nervous anxiety, constipation, menstrual cramps, and even headaches.

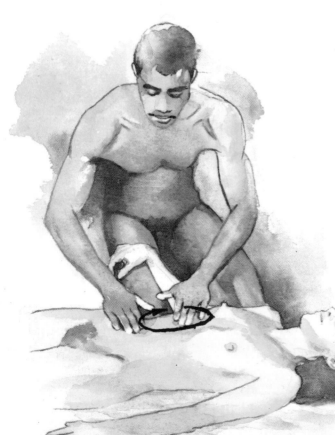

Starting the movement

Think of the palms of your hands as receptacles for a burning star. Warm your hands by rubbing your palms together in a relaxed but vigorous way. Keep your shoulders low and relaxed, and feel the stars glowing hot.

Apply warm oil all over your partner's belly (see pp. 63-4). Kneeling at your partner's right side, place your right palm below the navel and your left palm above the navel.

Move both hands simultaneously in a clockwise circle around the navel. Cross your right hand over your left as you make the circle, as if you were turning a steering wheel.

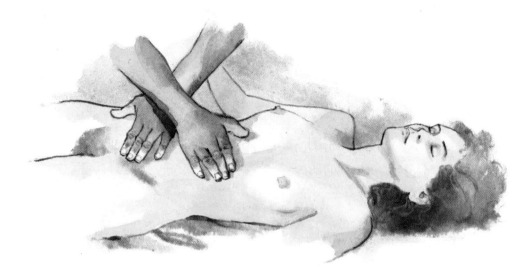

Completing the technique

As the heat increases, your pressure automatically lightens to a feather's weight. As you continue to circle, go lightly, as if you were rubbing gold leaf without tearing it. You will be moving your partner's finest and most profound energies. The sexual fire is ignited, stirred, and intensified.

The result of this is that a man may start to become erect; a woman may start to move her hips slowly from side to side. As these signs of excitement occur, stay centred, breathe slowly, and maintain the circular movement, without touching the genitals, until your intuition tells you to stop. Now rest your hands in the original starting position and let your energy settle.

Visualizing the energy
As you turn the abdominal flesh around in circles, you will feel heat growing in your hands. The massage ignites the sexual energy stored in the pelvic region. Stirring it in a clockwise circle increases its strength and temperature.

Working from your abdomen
Feel your own lower abdomen grow warm, and imagine that you are massaging your partner directly from there, using your hands as instruments for the flow of energy.

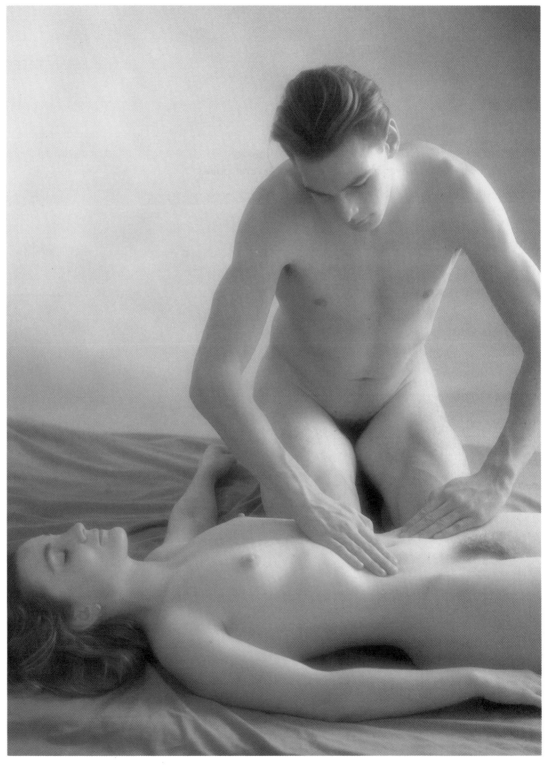

Building the Fire under the Stove (see pp. 138-9)

Resting on the Lower Abdomen

By this point in the massage sequence you have opened up a powerful current of energy down the mid-line of the body. In doing this, you have helped your partner to make the link between the upper, mental centres, and the lower, sexual centres (see p. 32).

This hold on the lower abdomen activates several points relating to the kidneys, which produce feelings of fear and anxiety when low in energy. Stimulating them enhances your partner's feelings of security. The technique usually induces a feeling of great safety and comfort, and at the same time stimulates sexual energy. Feeling secure in this region is crucial to your partner's full enjoyment of sexual stimulation.

Resting on the Lower Abdomen

Rest your left palm lightly on the lower abdomen, your fingers touching the top of the pubic bone. Visualize your palm and fingers making the lower abdomen spread out. Allow your body heat to flow through your palm in order to heat up the area that you are touching. Maintain this hold for about 30 seconds.

Pounding the Doors of the Crimson Palace

Pounding the Doors of the Crimson Palace brings the attention to the heart centre again (see p. 101), this time to free up inhibitions. The technique loosens your partner's inner "judge" who likes to control, and inhibits fun. As a result, your partner will feel light-hearted and ready for more stimulation.

This technique taken in isolation will also help respiratory problems and release tension from the chest.

Pounding the Doors

Form loose fists, then slowly and lightly percuss (see p. 78) the centre of the breastbone between the breasts, with regular, alternating beats. Keep the tempo steady and maintain a light and even pressure. Let each beat feel as if it is penetrating through to your partner's back.

Maintain this movement for about one minute. Keep your shoulders, elbows, and wrists completely relaxed; otherwise you will transmit stiffness.

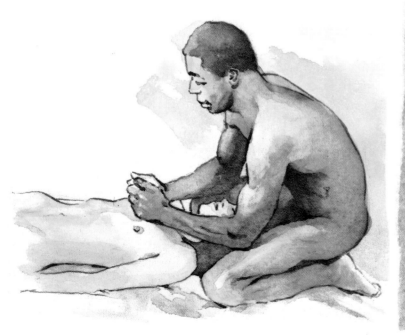

The release of passion
Performed as part of the massage sequence, this technique may release powerful childhood feelings of passion that might have been blocked for years. Childlike feelings of playful adventurousness are prerequisite to a healthy sex life. After all, sex is meant to be fun. Your partner may feel a fizzing sensation once you have stopped, signalling the release of energy.

Harmonizing Fire and Water Part I

This powerful movement collects and transports the body's energy to the genital region with force, and the sexual response can be surprisingly strong.

The technique is especially useful for people who have great fear of sex. It engenders feelings of self acceptance and confidence. It is often used to help treat depressive emotions.

Moving the energy

Place your palms lightly on the centre of your partner's breastbone. Very slowly push down toward the pubic bone, leading with your finger pads (see the Flat Hand Stroke, p. 80).

At the pubic bone, separate your hands over the hip bones. Pull up the sides to the armpits and around the breasts to the centre. Ask your partner to breathe in as you come up, and out as you go down.

The cycle lasts about 30 seconds. Repeat it at an even speed and pressure for about five minutes.

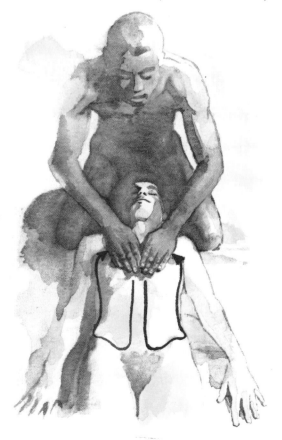

Harmonizing Fire and Water

The chest is the home of the element Fire (see p. 25) which instills passion into consciousness. The lower abdomen is the home of the element Water, which instills vitality into consciousness. When the two are blended, harmonized, and transported around the body, you feel a tidal wave of warm, nurturing love moving through you.

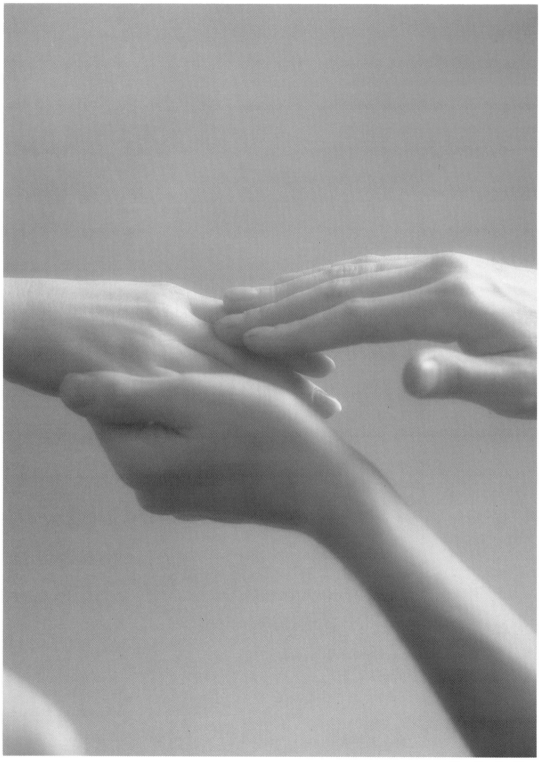

Greeting the Five

Greeting the Five

This technique stimulates the sexual force in the chest and upper body by working on the energy channel of the Heart Protector in the arm. Used as part of the whole sequence, the effects are considerable.

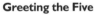

Greeting the Five
Take hold of your partner's hand in one of yours, with the back of their hand facing up. Stroke back and forth along the backs of the fingers between the hand and the first knuckle. Work very slowly and very lightly, from the little finger to the thumb.

Spend about 30 seconds on each finger. Then move to the other side and repeat this on the other hand.

It is vital to maintain your focus and sensitivity while performing this miniature movement.

Peaks and valleys
This may appear to be painstaking and minimalist when compared to Harmonizing Fire and Water (see p. 143), but it is this contrast that leads sexual energy through valleys, peaks, and plateaus (see pp. 84-5).

Leading the Fire

This technique helps to relieve the tension that accumulates from trying to control life. The strain of trying to control events manifests in the hands. This is because they are the body's main tool and point of interaction with the outside world. By releasing tension in the hands, you will relax your partner's attempts to control events, and increase the level of surrender to the rest of the massage.

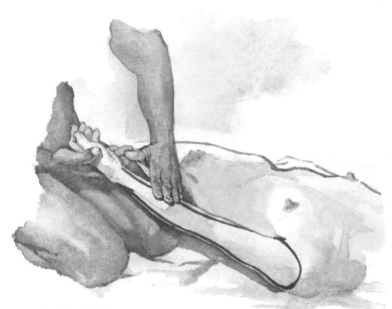

Leading the Fire

Take command of your partner's arm by taking one hand in yours. With your partner's palm facing up, run your fingertips from the middle of the palm, up the mid-line of the soft inside of the arm, lingering for a brief moment in the elbow crease, and then up into the armpit.

Continue by running your fingers over the front of the shoulder, then down the middle of the outside of the arm to the knuckles. Ask your partner to breathe in as your hand goes up, and out as the stroke follows downward.

Repeat the cycle slowly and lightly for about one minute on each arm.

Working on the consciousness

Leading the Fire maintains the level of sexual energy on a plateau (see p. 84-5), in suspension, ready for an acceleration. At the same time it leads the Fire energy to mingle with Water at a deeper level than does Harmonizing Fire and Water (see p. 143). It also calms the nerves and augments the now rapidly altering state of your partner's consciousness.

Approaching the Crimson Palace

Approaching the Crimson Palace dispels any block of energy in the armpit, and this in turn greatly increases the overall flow of vitality.

The movement also eases tension in the upper chest and opens up the heart energy in the Crimson Palace. These points accumulate tension in response to pleasure as well as pain. Leading the Fire (see facing page) may cause a small amount of tension to build up here. You may find that your partner unconsciously blocks and prevents sexual pleasure entering the body from the arms.

Dispelling energy blocks
Place your thumb in the centre of the armpit, and your fingers on the pectoral muscles at the upper sides of the chest. Squeezing your fingers and thumb together firmly, circle the thumb in the armpit and the fingers on the pectoral muscle.

Continue this for about one minute, then move to the other side of your partner and repeat, using the other hand for the squeezing motion.

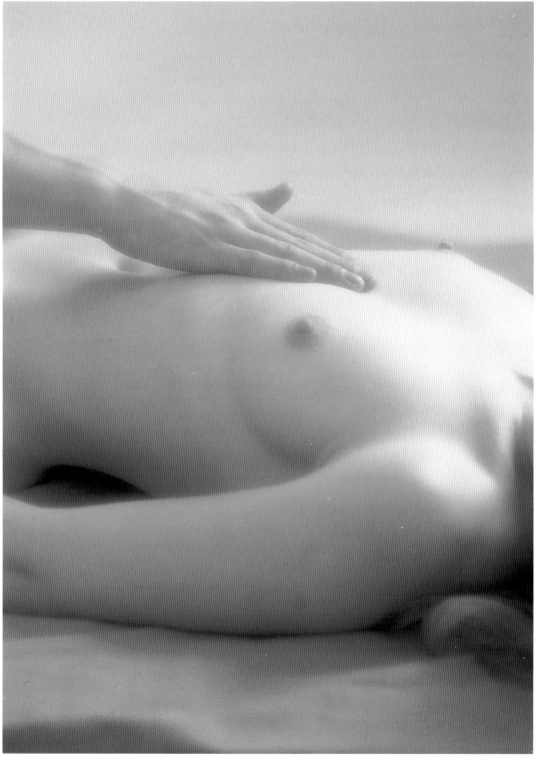

Opening the Doors of the Crimson Palace

Opening the Doors of the Crimson Palace

This movement on the chest has a direct effect on the heart centre, or Crimson Palace, opening it and releasing feelings of euphoria and love. It engenders trust and prepares the way for the first genital contact. It also raises the level of joy and humour and will often lead to laughter.

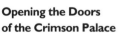

**Opening the Doors
of the Crimson Palace**
Place the finger pads of your right hand on the centre of your partner's breastbone. Move the skin in a slow, even, clockwise circle, against the breastbone. Continue in this way for about 30 seconds.

Working on the chest
It may seem strange to the western mind that so many techniques for sexual enhancement focus on the chest. However, it is only through feelings of warmth in the chest, combined with genital excitation, that sexual union can feel complete.

Harmonizing Fire and Water Part II

This technique will exponentially multiply sexual energy and it is important to restrain from any form of sexual contact at this point other than the massage. To do otherwise would be like taking the cake from the oven before it is thoroughly baked.

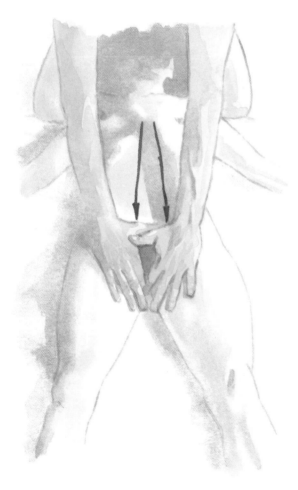

Starting the movement

As with Harmonizing Fire and Water Part I (see p. 143), place your hands on the centre of the chest. Using the Flat Hand Stroke (see p. 80), slowly move them down toward the pubic bone with an even speed and pressure. Instead of stopping there, continue down between the legs to the perineum.

On a woman (see left) your fingers will pass lightly over the clitoris and the labia, which will noticeably raise levels of sexual excitation. If you are working on a man, see the illustration at the bottom of the facing page.

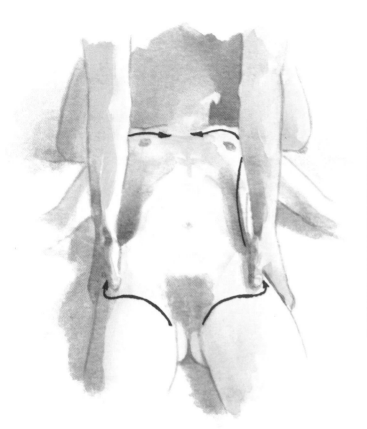

Completing the technique
From the perineum, part your hands and pull them over the tops of the thighs and up along the sides of the body (see the Pulling Stroke, p. 82). Allow your thumbs to brush the nipples gently as you bring your hands over the breasts to meet again in the centre of the breastbone. This comprises one cycle.

Repeat the cycle for up to three minutes, gradually allowing your hands to make more contact with the nipples as you pass over the breasts. This further stimulates the nipples.

Working on a man
On a man, you pass each side of the penis and scrotum, which may induce an erection. Continue down between the legs and over the perineum. Then continue as for a woman.

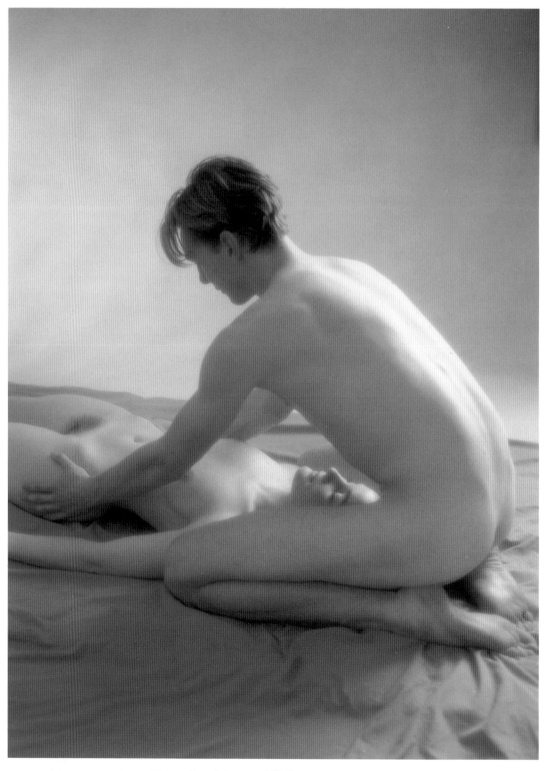

Harmonizing Fire and Water Part II (see pp. 150-1)

Ascending the Steps of the Jade Pagoda

This movement works on the upper back region from which the ego likes to control the body and inhibit natural, healthy sexual movements lower down. The technique helps to reduce that control, heals your partner of muscular tension - which is sometimes produced by shortening the upper back to deny the full, ecstatic pleasure of orgasm - and enables the hips to receive energy from the upper parts. The movement also helps to relieve headaches, stiff necks, and rigid attitudes.

Starting the movement

Place the palms of your hands together and think of them as a pillow filled with golden feathers.

Now face the palms upward and reach down under each side of your partner's upper back. Pull up over the spine and on to the back of the skull, with a slow, firm, but gentle stroke. Allow your finger pads to make contact with each vertebra, as your hands travel upward.

The Emperor and the Ego

At the very top of the Jade Pagoda sits the Emperor's Supreme Command of the Realm. He requires the spinal column and supporting muscles to be supple and relaxed, in order to receive instructions from the Emperor in the heart and to send back information to the lower parts of the body.

The Ego, usurper of the realm, is always trying to seal off the heights of the Jade Pagoda by creating unnecessary tension in these muscles. This hinders the flow of energy, blood, nerve impulses, and information between the control tower, or Cave of the Original Spirit, in the centre of the brain (see p. 113), and the rest of the bodily realm below.

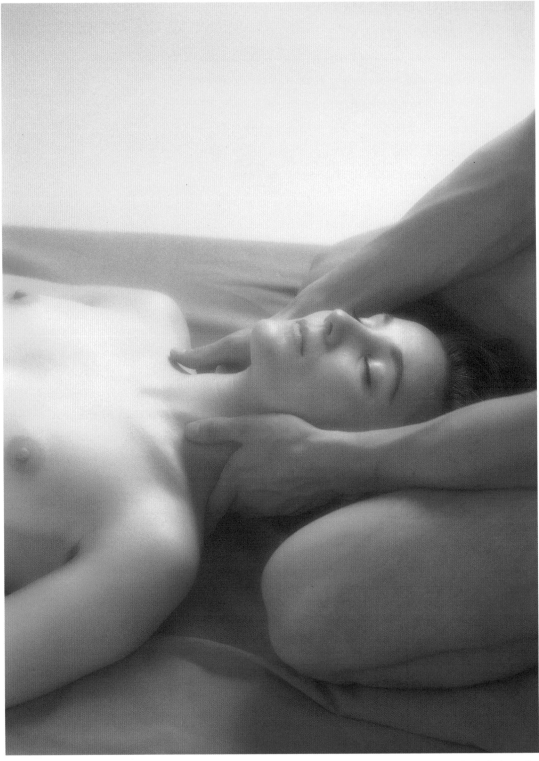

Ascending the Steps of the Jade Pagoda

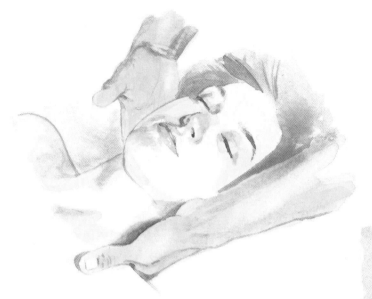

*(Ascending the Steps
of the Jade Pagoda contd.)*

Completing the technique

On your second massage stroke, pull up the muscles on either side of the spine. Each time you repeat this technique make sure that your own upper back area stays relaxed and soft, and that your breath is flowing smoothly. Let the movement start from deep inside your pelvic area, as if you are massaging your partner from your pelvis, and your hands are merely the instruments.

After about one minute, continue the massage by pulling up one side of the neck at a time. This will help to ease the uneven levels of tension on each side of the neck that result from postural imbalance.

Visualize, and ask your friend to visualize, the release of past pain and burden with every stroke. This allows your hands to find their own natural level of pressure, just as water finds its own level.

End this massage with your hands cupped underneath the skull base, like the pillow filled with golden down, gently pulling on the head and so lengthening the spine. Use your intuition to tell you the right time to let your hands rest.

Allow your energies to settle.

Reactions in the body

Several reactions are likely to occur. You may witness a relaxation of the entire body, as if your partner has just remembered him or herself as a Divine Being.

The hips and genital areas might seem to open up, as the Supreme Commander begins to feel more secure.

If you have been sensitive and sensually receptive yourself, you will notice your partner react to the contact by hip movements, erection of the nipples or penis, and other signs of sexual excitation.

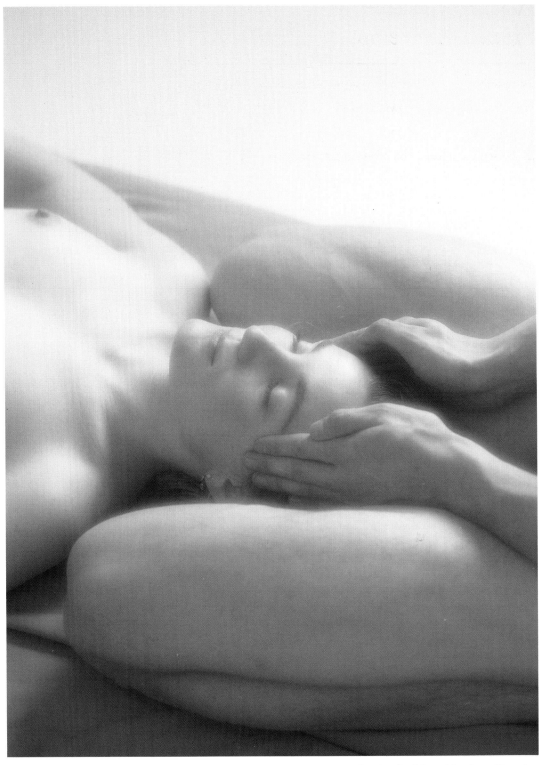

Resting Position - Hands on Temples

Resting Position - Hands on Temples

By resting your hands on your partner's temples, you bring the level of sexual energy down from the peak to a plateau level - (see pp. 84-5) and give your partner's body time to assimilate all the sensual information given so far. From here the intention is to climb again to a new peak.

Resting on the temples

Rest your fingertips on your partner's temples. Feel as if your fingers are melting into your partner's head. Watch the eyes as they appear to sink back in their sockets. This is a sign that your partner is sinking into a deeper internal consciousness.

Maintain this light hold for up to one minute, allowing your own energy to settle.

Resting Position - Inner Ankles

This technique provides a plateau upon which the sexual energy can settle. These plateaus are as essential as are the peaks in building the erotic force. They give your partner time to assimilate the new sensations. This leads to a great feeling of security, which is necessary in order to experience a total orgasm. Resting before continuing with the techniques that follow adds drama to the next technique, Flying on the Land (see facing page), which accelerates considerably the build up of erotic force.

Holding the inner ankles

From the resting position on the temples (see p. 157), move down to your partner's feet. Place your partner's legs about two feet apart, and hold your palms on the inner ankle bones in a firm and reassuring way, fingers facing inward. Feel as if you are taking command of the legs.

Holding the legs open in this way provides a moment of suspense, with your partner in a state of lust and vulnerability. The genitals are exposed to your view, and it is important to let your energies settle and stay with the massage sequence if you are to facilitate the next peak experience.

Maintain this firm hold, feeling into the ankles, for about 30 seconds.

Flying on the Land

This movement stimulates the earth energies and lends a feeling of grounding and stability to the sexual energy. It engenders a feeling of safety and security in your partner, ready for you to make the next genital contact.

The name of the movement, Flying on the Land, describes the sensation of floating above the ground that you would feel if you were to walk after receiving this part of the massage.

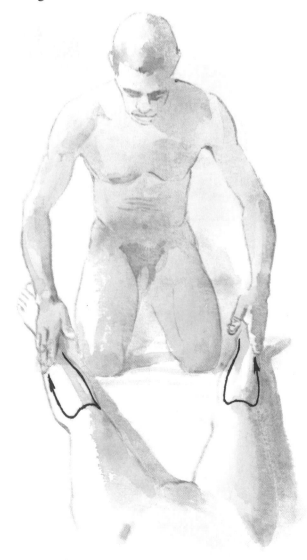

Flying on the Land
From the resting position at the inner ankles (see p. 158), slowly push your palms up the inside of the shinbones to the knees, then up and over the front of the knees. Pull down the outside of the shinbones (see left) to the outer ankle and cross over to the inside ankle again. This comprises one cycle and can be repeated for about one minute. Ask your partner to breathe in as your hands go up and out as they come down.

As you work up the leg, feel as if you are leading a tidal wave of energy. Just before you turn your hands over the knees, make a small pushing, or flicking gesture with your fingers as if to encourage the wave to travel all the way up to the genitals.

Awakening the Dragon

This movement around the inner and outer thighs contacts the earth energies of the Stomach and Spleen Channels. It is used in the treatment of vaginitis, frigidity, and inability to have an erection. It also strengthens the blood, which improves anaemia. It increases motivation and enthusiasm for life.

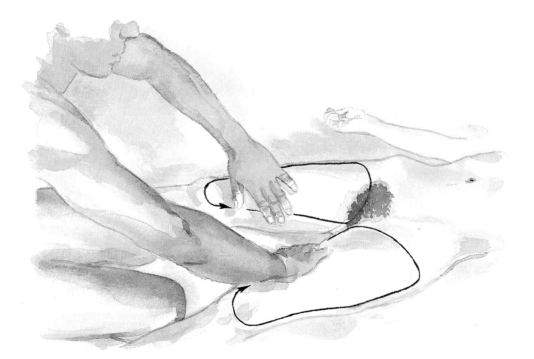

Awakening the Dragon

Visualize your palms as magnets that conduct the energy of the earth. Rest one palm on each of your partner's knees, and feel the energy flow into your partner's body. Now let your hands travel slowly up the inside of the thighs to meet at the perineum. Then part them, and move your finger pads along the inguinal groove between the leg and body to the hip bones.

From the hip bones, pull your palms down the outer thighs to the knees. Then circle them over the knees and start the whole movement again.

As you notice your partner's level of sexual excitation increase - in the male by erection of the penis, in the female by an opening and moistening of the labia - lighten your pressure until you are hardly touching the skin. Your intuition will tell you when to stop. Rest your hands at the perineum, palms resting on the thighs. Let your energy settle.

The Spleen Channel

Just above the knee, on the inner thigh, is a focus of energy on the Spleen Channel, called the Sea of Vigour, or Sea of Blood. The Channel conducts invigorating Earth energy (see The Five Elements, p. 25) to the genital region, supplying the foundation for the sexual vitality in the lower abdomen.

The Stomach Channel

The outer thigh, especially just above the knee, contacts the Stomach Channel, which is also connected to the Earth element. But the spleen and stomach pathways take different directions: the Spleen Channel conducts Earth energy deep into the body's core and eventually to the spleen itself, whereas the Stomach Channel guides energy that has been refined and processed by the spleen to the outer layers of the body and the digestive organs.

The Stomach Channel energy is responsible for enthusiasm and strong motivation for daily activities. By guiding the circulation of its elemental Earth energies, you strengthen sexual drive and sustaining power, and increase longevity and animal vigour.

The movement harmonizes your inner, sexual being with your outer, motivated being. It also strengthens the legs, which helps the lower back and spine; the hips become more open and relaxed. General energy and motivation levels increase.

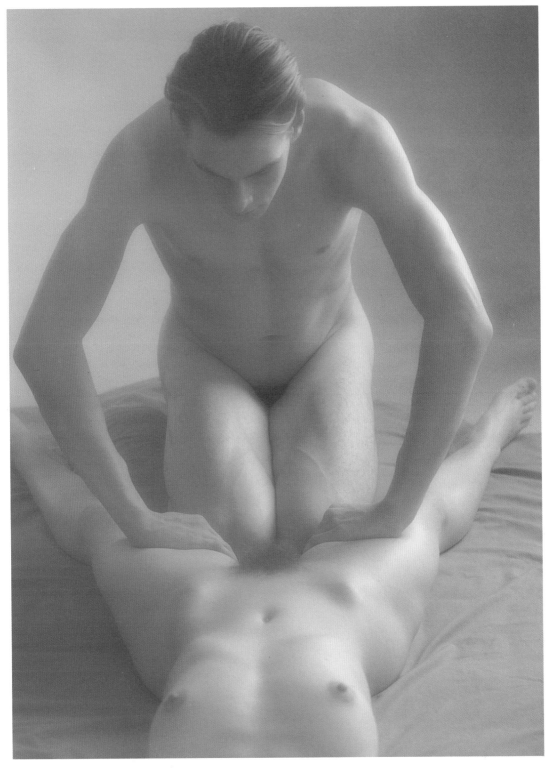

Awakening the Dragon (see p. 160)

Opening the Gate of Trust - for Women

This technique brings sexual energy to a great height, and must not be regarded as merely a sophisticated form of masturbation. As well as preparing your partner for the increasing levels of sexual energy, this massage balances all the energy of the body and tones the whole organism.

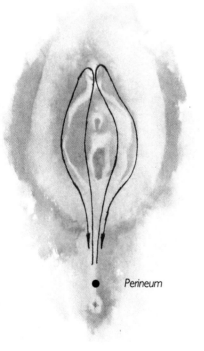

Perineum

Opening the Gate of Trust

Continue as if you were completing another cycle of Awakening the Dragon (see p. 160-1 and facing page). Let your hands travel up the inner thighs to meet at the perineum. Instead of separating them at this point, gently move your fingertips up between the outer lips of the vagina, over the clitoris. Then separate your hands over the hood of the clitoris, and stroke down around the outer lips of the vagina, to meet again at the perineum.

Always stroke slowly and lightly, as if stroking gold leaf without allowing it to tear.

Continue to stroke up between the vaginal lips, over the clitoris, then down each side, around the outer vaginal lips to the perineum. Repeat this cycle around the vaginal lips for about two minutes.

Opening the Gate of Trust - for Men

This technique is the equivalent of the sequence for women (see p. 163). Such a highly sensual movement will increase desire for deeper sexual contact but it is unlikely to cause ejaculation. In order to benefit from the full effect of the technique, it is important to restrain from leaving the massage sequence at this point. The movement has the same effect of toning the entire energy system for men as it does for women. For men, it also greatly reduces the tendency to premature ejaculation.

Two methods
There are two ways to perform this part of the massage on a man, depending on whether or not he has an erection.

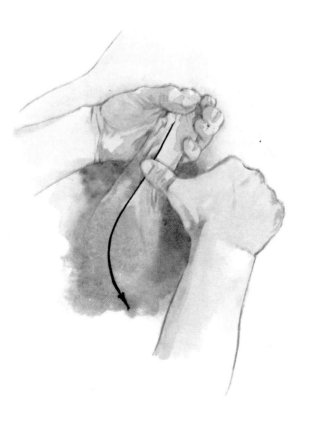

Non-erect sequence

If your partner does not have an erection at the start of the massage, use the thumb and forefinger of your left hand (unless you are left-handed) and expose your partner's scrotum by gently lifting up the penis. Rest your hand on the pubic bone, with the penis in your palm. With your other hand cup the scrotum very gently.

Rest in this position for a few seconds. The warmth of your touch allows energy to penetrate deep into the Gate of Trust.

Keeping your right hand gently cupped, stroke upward with your thumb until you reach your other hand (see left). Hold the penis cupped between both hands for a few seconds, then, lightening your touch, stroke down from the scrotum until you reach your partner's perineum with your right hand. Keep your touch light and focus your awareness on this hand. Do not squeeze the testicles. Take your time, there is no hurry.

Erect sequence

If your partner has an erection, start this massage by holding the glans of the penis lightly between thumb and forefinger, with the back of your hand on his abdomen, so as to maintain the penis in the erect position.

Using the thumb of the other hand, stroke up the median line of the scrotum and then up the underside of the penis to the tip. Then use the thumb and forefinger to stroke down each side of the penis and around the outside of each testicle, to meet again at the perineum.

This comprises one cycle and can be continued for about two minutes.

Turning the Fire - for Women

By this point in the massage sequence, all the energies of the body are highly stimulated. Having completed the massage techniques so far, and manipulated the energy flow in such a sophisticated manner, the effect of this one can be startling. Sexual energy will rise to a new level and create a strongly altered state of consciousness.

If your partner spontaneously experiences orgasm at this point, which often happens, that is fine, but do not let it be the goal of this particular exercise.

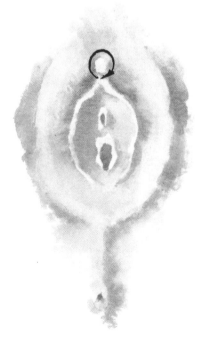

Turning the Fire
Move your fingertips between the lips of the vagina up to the clitoris in the same way as you would to complete another cycle of Opening the Gate of Trust for Women (see p. 163). Then, with thumb or fingerpad, press lightly on the clitoris, as if to make an indentation in dough. Now start circling the skin directly surrounding the clitoris, using a clockwise direction. Continue this for about three minutes.

Turning the Fire - for Men

Turning the Fire has a highly strengthening effect on the sexual energy and the body as a whole. It is unlikely to cause ejaculation, but will build the desire for close union. If you wish to experience the full effect of the massage, restrain yourself from deviating from the sequence at this point.

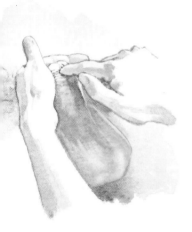

Non-erect sequence

If your partner does not have an erection, stroke up the median line of the penis with your thumb. As you reach the top of the penis, change to use the finger pad of your index finger to massage very gently the point on the median line that lies on the underside of the penis, where the foreskin is attached to the glans. Use a clockwise circular motion.

Erect sequence

If your partner has an erection, continue stroking up the penis. When you arrive at the glans, take the penis into your left hand (if you are right-handed) as if you were holding a wand, and pull back the foreskin as far as possible. Using your thumb or pad of your right index finger, softly massage around the outside perimeter of the glans in a clockwise circle.

Continue this for about three minutes, with light, even pressure and slow, even pace.

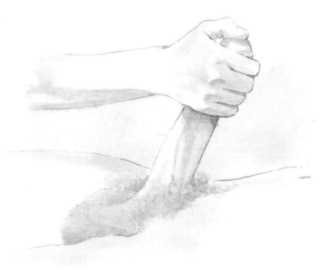

Harmonizing the Whole

This last movement in the sequence connects and harmonizes all the body's energies. The technique combines all the movements of the sequence so far, including Flying on the Land (see p. 159), Awakening the Dragon (see pp. 160-2), Leading the Fire (see p. 146), and Harmonizing Fire and Water (see pp. 143 and 150-2). This combined stroke intensifies the energy in the body; by this time it is highly charged with sexual force.

Starting the movement

Stand with your feet level with your partner's thighs, knees bent. Reach down between your legs, so that your fingertips contact as closely as possible to your partner's inner ankles.

With a gentle, sweeping motion, run your fingertips lightly up the inside of each leg to the perineum. Part your hands over the hips and run them lightly up the sides of the body, over the front of the shoulders.

Completing the technique

Continue by running the hands lightly down the outside of the arms to the hands. From the hands, run up the insides of the arms to the armpits, over the breasts to the centre of the breastbone, then down to the pubic bone. Now separate your hands and run them down the outsides of the legs to the outer ankle.

This comprises one cycle. Repeat it for about one minute.

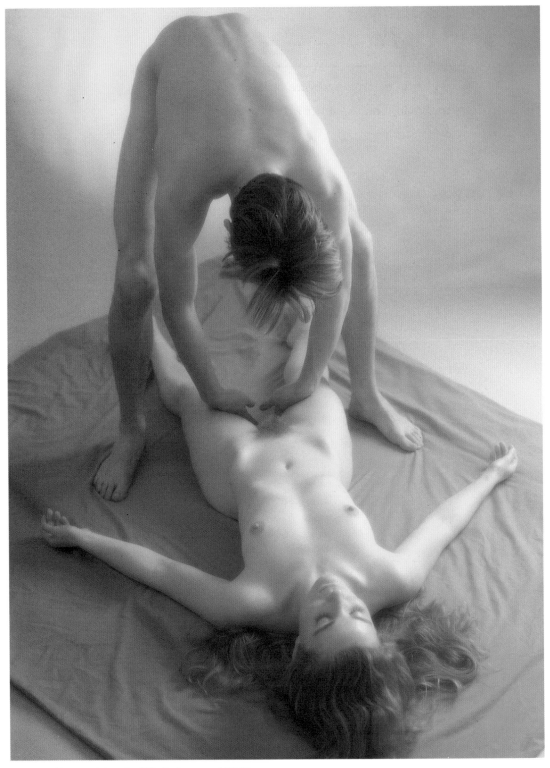

Harmonizing the Whole (see pp. 168-9)

Resting Position - Holding the Pelvis

This is the last position in the front sequence of the massage. The hold feels very healing and engenders a deep sense of trust and gratitude in your partner.

Deep contact through the palms

Ask your partner to lift their hips, so that you can slide your hand between their legs and under the sacrum, fingers pointing up along the spine.

Then ask your partner to lower back down gently on to your palm. Keeping your hand in contact with the skin, move the flesh over the sacrum, pulling downward, toward the heels. This creates a stretch along the spine.

Place your other palm, fingers toward the head, so that the heel of your hand is resting on the perineum, and your fingers either under the penis, or on the pubic bone.

Maintain this deep contact through your palms for 30 seconds or so, allowing your body heat to flow through your hands into the genital region of your partner.

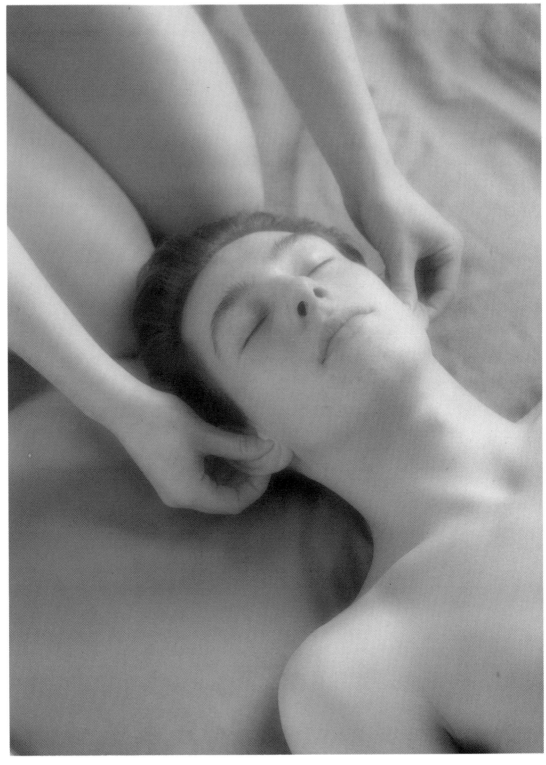

Watering the Flowers of the Kidneys

FINAL SEQUENCE

The following, final techniques are an aid to ending the massage in a totally harmonized way, feeling grounded, refreshed, and regenerated.

If you choose to engage in sexual activity now, complete the remaining techniques afterwards.

Watering the Flowers of the Kidneys

According to Taoist belief, the ears are the outward flower of the kidneys. By massaging the ears all over, you will be stimulating the flow of "Ancestral" energy from the kidneys (see p. 33), throughout the entire organism. This strengthens the kidneys, which helps to overcome anxiety. It also raises vitality levels, and engenders a feeling of optimism.

Watering the Flowers of the Kidneys
Place your fingers behind the ears, and use your thumbs to massage into the ears with a small circular motion. Work round every nook and cranny until the ears are hot and slightly red. Continue for about 30 seconds.

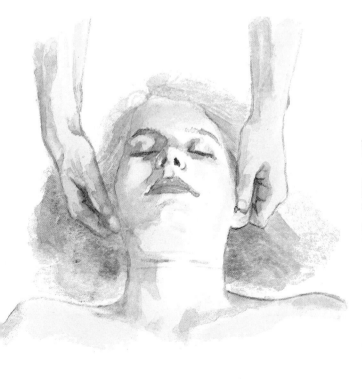

Fetal resemblance
If you project the shape of an inverted fetus onto the ear, you can then link points on the ear to major energy centres in the body and work on them through massage. For example, if you stimulate the point on the ear corresponding with the area of the heart of the fetus, this will send energy to the heart.

Opening the Doors to the Mysterious Passageway

This technique increases the flow of energy along the Mysterious Passageway (see right) to the pituitary gland (see facing page), and on to the sexual glands, preparing for a huge stimulation of sexual energy - the Original Fire at the Gate of the Spine.

The movement calls together all the spiritual, mental, and emotional bodies, and invites them to congregate as one, centred around the spinal axis.

At the same time, you will soothe away headaches, clear the sinuses, energize the eyes, and relax the entire skull. Your partner will feel centred, empty of mental turmoil, and receptive.

The Mysterious Passageway
The Mysterious Passageway leads backward through the mid-brain region, past the pituitary gland, to the top of the spinal column, into the Cave of the Original Spirit, where the Original and Supreme Consciousness of our Universe lives and from where it directs the true actions of the being.

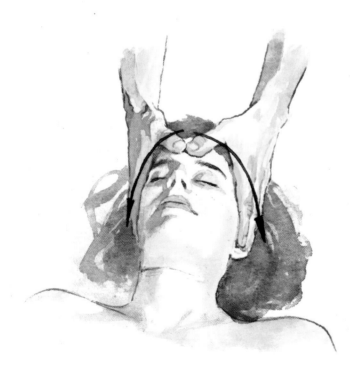

Starting the movement
Rest your fingers on the sides of the head, and gently position your thumbs on the middle of the forehead, just above the top line of the eyebrows. Slowly and deliberately, guide each thumb outward to the temples. Do not stretch the skin, but allow your thumb pads to furrow through the brow. Bring your thumbs back from the end of the brow to the centre of the forehead.

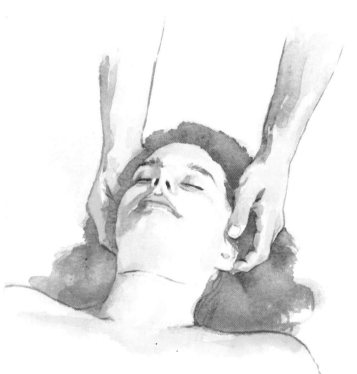

Completing the technique

As you repeat this movement, think of yourself smoothing all unnecessary mental activity, delusions, and worries, outward to the temples. By smoothing your partner's mental stress, all the negative energy can escape into the macrocosm to be recycled into fresh mental energy.

When you instinctively feel this surplus energy has been released, visualize your movement opening up two sliding doors to reveal the Mysterious Passageway.

While you are doing this massage, ask your partner to imagine the space between and behind the eyes as a comforting and safe night sky.

It may take only three strokes to achieve the desired state, or it might take thirty-three. Your intuition will guide you when to stop. Rest your thumbs and fingers at the original position. Breathe deeply and let your energy settle.

The pituitary gland

Along the Mysterious Passageway sits the pituitary gland. Its link with the sexual glands is well known. Together these have an influence in the reproductive and sexual spheres.

Mental activity spinning in the forebrain seriously hinders their combined function. The movement you are making calms the forebrain and stimulates the pituitary gland.

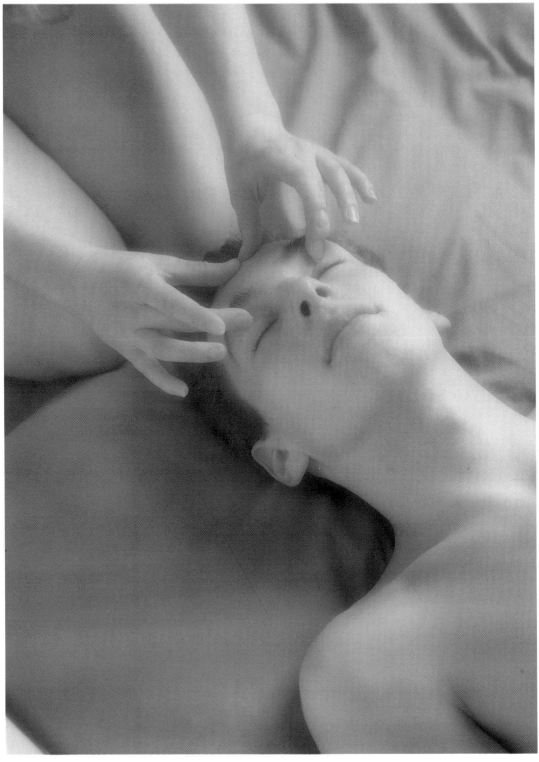

Orbiting the Sun and Moon

Orbiting the Sun and Moon

This technique brings the Yin and Yang energies into harmony. Its enhances the eyesight, relieves eye strain and migraine, and generally brightens your partner's outlook on life.

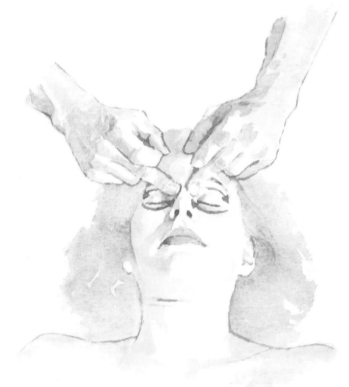

Orbiting the Sun and Moon

Rest your thumbs on your partner's forehead, and use your finger pads to move gently around the bony orbits that surround your partner's closed eyes. Move inward underneath the eyes to the inner comers, and then lift your fingers away and repeat the movement.

Use only light pressure. Let each orbit last a few seconds. Continue the movement for about one minute.

Yin, Yang, and the eyes
According to Taoist beliefs, the right eye is linked to the Yang energy of the sun - bright and revealing. The left eye is linked to the Yin energy of the moon - dark and veiled. The eyes are considered to be the two major points for gaining access to the Yin and Yang energies of the entire body.

Fuelling the Middle Burner

Smoothing tension away from the cheeks eases the digestive organs, or Middle Burner (see box, below right), and brightens your partner's disposition. The technique also helps to clear the sinuses, which may block during sexual activity or massage, due to errant kidney energy rushing upward.

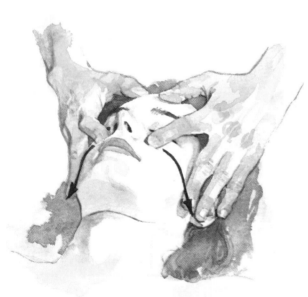

Fuelling the Middle Burner
Place your thumbs at the middle of the forehead and use the pads of your forefingers to massage from the sides of the nose, just below the eyes, over the fleshiest parts of the cheeks, to the corners of the jawbone, below the ears. Use an even, moderate pressure. Repeat for about one minute.

The Middle Burner

The cheeks contact the energies of the gall bladder, spleen, stomach, pancreas, and liver - organs that are collectively known as the Middle Burner.

Digestive strain and stress create tension in the cheeks; this tension is exacerbated by the daily wearing of false smiles, frowns and by holding any expression for too long. As a result, tension in the cheeks affects the digestive organs.

Strengthening the Will

This massage on the chin strengthens the kidneys and so increases will power and resolve. The expression "chinless" describes being weak-willed - the opposite condition. Working on this area also strengthens the eyes, ears, and facial muscles.

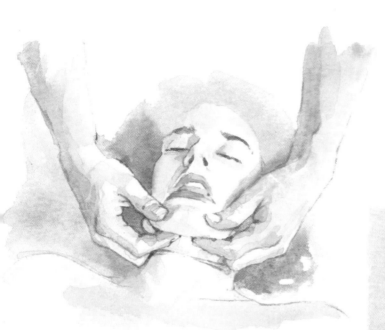

Strengthening the Will

Trace a line down from the corners of the mouth to the chinbone. Place your thumbs at the points where the line meets the chin, and your fingers underneath the chinbone.

Circle your thumbs in outwardly directed circles, moving the skin over the chinbone. Continue with moderate pressure and even tempo for approximately 30 seconds.

Kidney energy

Kidney energy is responsible for your will power; this technique enhances your kidney energy and so helps to strengthen your partner's will and resolve.

Grasping the Jaw

The jaw region is a storehouse of old resentments, unexpressed anger, and unshed tears. This gentle technique frees the jaw area from unnecessary muscular tension, and so releases these stagnant emotions.

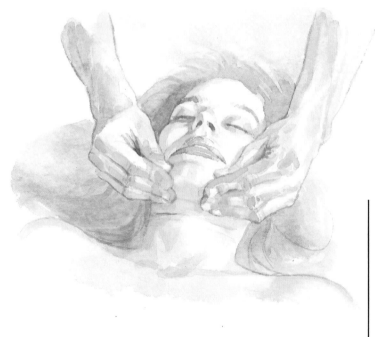

Grasping the Jaw

With your fingers poised under your partner's chin, slowly pull along the line of the jawbone, toward each ear. When you reach the ear, return to the starting position and repeat.

Each stroke should last about 10 seconds. Continue with light pressure for about one minute.

Regular practice will strengthen your partner's levels of tolerance toward other people's shortcomings.

Removing the Mask

If the eyes are considered to be the mirrors of the soul, then the face is the mirror of the personality.

This massage technique on the face has the effect of smoothing away the mask that your personality creates (see box, below right). It engenders a feeling of deep peace and a willingness to literally "face" the world anew.

Removing the Mask
Place your palms over your partner's face, your fingers pointing toward the navel, one palm on either side of the nose. Slowly and deliberately, spread the face by moving your hands outward to the sides of the head.

Maintain moderate pressure and even tempo as you repeat this movement for up to one minute. Your partner will feel reborn.

The mask of personality
The word personality derives from the Greek word "persona", meaning mask. Behind the mask lies the Cave of the Original Spirit, the place from which your immortal self observes day-to-day reality (see p. 113). It is perfectly fitting to wear a mask. However, like any actor, it is essential to remove it from time to time, so that the spirit can gaze freely at the world.

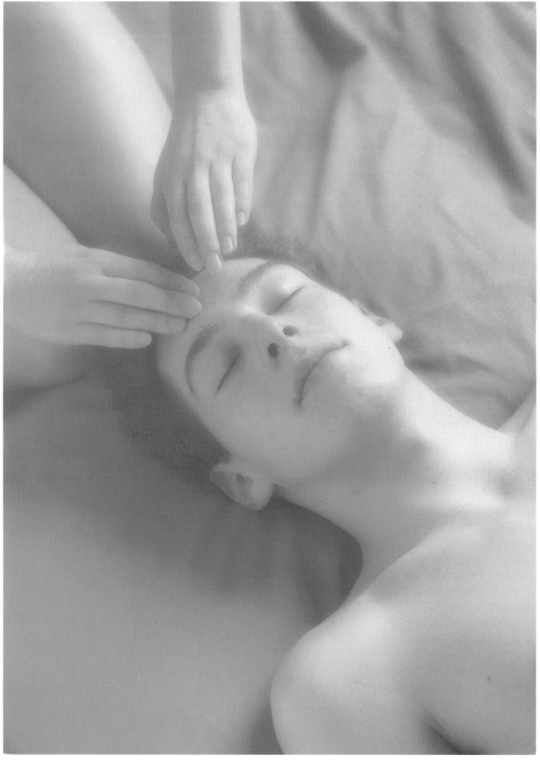

Pounding the Door of the Mysterious Passageway

Pounding the Door of the Mysterious Passageway

Pounding the Door of the Mysterious Passageway refreshes the area surrounding the eyes and makes your partner wide awake, ready for life.

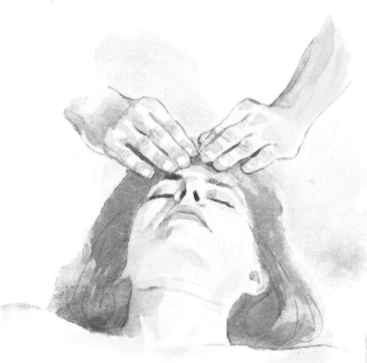

Pounding the Door
Using the pads of your fingers on both hands, percuss (see p. 78) the area in the middle of the forehead, up to two inches above the space between the eyebrows. Use an even tempo and maintain a light, steady drum roll with even pressure for about one minute.

Back to consciousness
This technique opens the Door to the Mysterious Passageway (see p. 174) and allows free access of vision to the Original Spirit within. It is a powerful way to bring your partner back into a normal state of consciousness.

Final Resting Position - Forehead

Stimulating the point in the middle of the forehead just above the line of the eyebrows is one of the most effective techniques for drawing together all the scattered parts of your partner's consciousness and energy into a unified whole.

Having led your partner through the innermost senses and intimate feelings, stimulating the point is akin to throwing the master switch for spiritual renewal. It is a simple technique, but one through which a Taoist master can heal the most complex conditions.

Healing light

Visualize the forefinger of your right hand emitting a powerful line of white light. Place your forefinger gently on the middle of the forehead, just above the line of the eyebrows. Picture the light from your fingers penetrating the brain, cleansing and renewing the Cave of the Original Spirit (see p. 174). Keep the pressure of your touch as light as a small bird resting on your palm. Maintain the hold for about one minute, then very slowly withdraw your finger.

The Happy Point

In Taoist medicine the entrance to the Mysterious Passageway, which leads back to the Cave of the Original Spirit, is often called "The Happy Point".

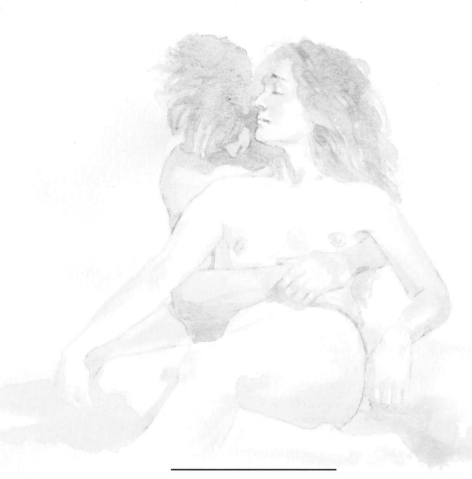

This completes the massage sequence.

At this time hold your partner in a loving embrace.

Take some minutes together for quiet contemplation.

Allow your breath, energy, and mental activity to settle.

It is advisable to wash and shake your hands.

This is a ritualistic trigger for your mind to release any

negative energy that you may have collected

from your partner's energy field.

Treating Common Ailments

Regular repetition of the complete Taoist sexual massage sequence harmonizes the entire body and mind. You can also use selected techniques alone or in combination, with the more specific aim of bringing improvements to a whole range of ailments, as shown on the facing page.

Regular repetition of the recommended techniques for five minutes every morning for one week will bring results. The resulting improvements will depend on the skill and sensitivity of the masseur and the receptivity of the person being massaged.

Although many of these conditions may appear to be unrelated to the realm of sexual massage, they are typical of the problems that are produced by blocked energy in the body, and which can block full sexual enjoyment.

Use these techniques alone, or to complement other styles of treatment such as acupuncture or herbology. They are not intended to replace conventional medical treatment, but can be a useful adjunct to it.

Shortened massage sequence
The full massage sequence (see pp. 94-184) takes about one hour for one partner to perform.

If you want to give and receive a massage in the same session, or if you do not have enough time for the full-length sequence, try the following, shortened version. Incorporate any additional parts of the sequence, according to the time you have available.

Back sequence
Supporting the Column, Parts 1 and 2 (pp. 108-9 and 118-20); Leading the Water (pp. 124-5)

Front sequence
Harmonizing Fire and Water, Parts 1 and 2 (pp. 143 and 150-2); Awakening the Dragon (pp. 160-2)

Ailments Chart

Anxiety attacks	Pounding the Rear Door of the Crimson Palace Harmonizing Fire & Water, Part 1	**Hypertension**	Supporting the Column, Part 1 Flying on the Land Harmonizing Fire & Water, Part 1
Back pain	Supporting the Column, Part 1	**Impotence**	Supporting the Column, Part 1 Pounding the Gate of the Spine Harmonizing Fire & Water, Parts 1 & 2 Leading the Water
Constipation	Harmonizing Fire & Water, Part 1		
Depression	Opening the Doors to the Mysterious Passageway Harmonizing Fire & Water, Part 1 Jiggling the Column	**Indigestion**	Harmonizing Fire & Water, Part 1
		Insomnia	Opening the Mysterious Passageway Leading the Fire Harmonizing Fire & Water, Part 1 Pounding the Rear Door of the Crimson Palace
Ejaculation - premature	Supporting the Column, Part 1 Jiggling the Column Awakening the Dragon Leading the Water		
Energy - improving low energy	Awakening the Dragon Supporting the Column, Part 1 Building the Fire under the Stove	**Legs - tiredness**	Flying on the Land Awakening the Dragon
		Menstruation - irregular	Flying on the Land Awakening the Dragon
Eye strain	Orbiting the Sun & Moon	**Neck pain**	Ascending the Steps of the Jade Pagoda
Frigidity	Harmonizing Fire & Water, Parts 1 & 2 Flying on the Land Leading the Fire Opening the Doors to the Mysterious Passageway	**Orgasm - inability to**	Resting position - Sacrum
		Respiratory problems	Pounding the Doors of the Crimson Palace
Headaches	Opening the Doors to the Mysterious Passageway	**Vaginismus**	Awakening the Dragon Leading the Water

Authors' Acknowledgements

Stephen Russell would like to acknowledge the role of patients, friends, and children in moving him to write this book. A particular thank-you goes to Steve Nakovitch for his invaluable help and support. Jürgen Kolb extends his thanks to his companion and friend, Karin Weisensel, for her support and advice. Thanks to her also for the Aphrodisia oil recipe on page 63.

Publisher's Acknowledgements

Gaia Books would like to thank Michelle Atkinson, Ann Chandler, Nina Gale, Sara Mathews, Katherine Pate, Gill Smith, and Susan Walby, for editorial and production work; Mary Warren for the index; Catriona Reid, Dave Reed, Peter Walby and Frances Zinc of FCP Design, for help with design and typesetting; Brian Edginton and Beehive Illustration for photographic assistance and illustrations.
    Thanks also to Melvin Ashong, Frank Kramer, Karen Snyder, and Karin Weisensel for modelling; and to Cocoa of Cheltenham for supplying materials.

Resources

It is not possible to recommend teachers or healers in Taoist sexual massage. Clubs and institutions contradict the spirit of freedom and individuality that is part of Taoism; trained Masters in sexology who heal or teach do not advertize. To find out more, you may contact Stephen Russell (author), c/o Gaia Books.

Further Reading

Chang, Jolan
The Tao of the Loving Couple
Penguin Books (US) 1983

Chuen, Lam Kam,
The Way of Energy
Gaia Books (UK), Simon & Schuster (US & Australia) 1991

Chungliang Al Huang
Embrace Tiger, Return to Mountain: The Essence of Tai Ji
Celestial Arts 1987

Da Liu
The Tao of Health and Longevity
Paragon House (US & UK) 1991

Jarmey, Chris and John Tindall
Acupressure for Common Ailments
Gaia Books (UK), Simon & Schuster (US), Angus & Robertson (Australia) 1991

Kirsta, Alix
The Book of Stress Survival
Unwin Hyman (UK), Simon & Schuster (US), Allen & Unwin (Australia & New Zealand) 1989

Lidell, Lucinda
The Book of Massage
Ebury Press (UK), Simon & Schuster (US) 1989

Lundberg, Paul
The Book of Shiatsu
Gaia Books (UK), Simon & Schuster (US and Australia) 1992

Mantak Chia and Michael Winn
Taoist Secrets of Love
Aurora Press Inc. 1984

Anand, Margo
The Art of Sexual Ecstasy
Jeremy P. Tarcher (US) 1989
Aquarian Press (UK) 1992

Palos, Stephen
The Chinese Art of Healing
Herder and Herder Inc. (US) 1971
Bantam (UK) 1972

Douglas, Nik and Penny Slinger
Sexual Secrets
Destiny Books (US) 1986
Arrow Books (UK) 1982

Index

Bold numerals refer to main entries; italic numerals refer to photographs

abdomen 33, 38, 50, 67, 73, 75, 97-8, 137, 139, 141
acupuncture 26, 75, 186
adrenalin 59
    see also kidney energy
advanced practice **38-41**
agreements 65
ailments
    Ailments Chart 187
    Treating Common Ailments 186
    see also under specific disorders
"Ancestral" life energy 33, 173
    see also Ching Chi
angina 111
Anima and Animus 51-2
animal vigour 161
anus 118, 126
anxiety 111, 141, 173, 187
Approaching the Crimson Palace **147**
armpits 95, 109, 146, 147, 169
Ascending the Steps of the Jade
    Pagoda **153-5**, *154*, 187
asthma 111
Awakening the Dragon **160-1**, *162*, 187
awareness 15, 32, 34, 48, 57, 65, 118, 143, 183-4
    altered states 34-6, 61, **65-7**, 74, 104, 146, 166

back pain 104, 105, 106, 112, 187
Back Sequence **101-29**
bladder 109
Bladder Channel **109**, 115, 123, 125,126
bladder disorders 112
blood circulation 45, 50, 65, 153
brain 32, 34, 36, 42, 43, 48, 66, 113, 123, 153, 184
    forebrain 175
    mid-brain region 32, 174
    upper brainstem 17
Breaking the Flow **134-5**, *136*
breathing 33, 50, 57, 65, **67**, 73, 74, 97, 135
    synchronization 74
    meditation 33, 67
Building the Fire under the Stove **138-9**, *140*, 187

cardiovascular system 116
cautions 5, 112
Cave of the Original Spirit 50, 113, 153, 174, 181, 184
centring 35, 74, 86, 174

Channel of Control 32, **103-7**, 126
Channel of Function 32, 126
channel pathways 73
channels (meridians) **26-9**, 33, 38, 126
    see also named types
chest 48, 95, 147, 149
Chi **26**, 30, 54 see also Ching Chi
child care 51
children and sexuality 45-7
chin 179
Chinese medicine and philosophy
    see under Taoism
Ching Chi (sexual energy) 26, 33
    see also sexual fire
chiropractic treatment 112
circling the sexual energies **34**, 42
circulation disorders 112
Climbing the Column **106-7**
clitoris 150, 163, 166
comfort 62, 71, 175
conception 33
condoms 62, 65
conflict 30, 45, 46, 51-4, 58
consciousness see awareness
constipation 138, 187
contraception 65
Creation 30, 43
Crimson Palace **101**, 111, 132

depression 47, 143, 187
diaphragm 50, 57, 97, 135, 137
digestive organs 135, 161, 178
disease resistance 115
Divine Energy centres **32**, 33, 36, 47
Divine Spirit and Law 38, 59
DNA 38

ears 173, 179
Earth 24-5
earth energy 160-1
ecstasy 11, 30, 35-6, 70
ego 153
ejaculation 42-3, 167, 187
    premature 124, 164, 187
electromagnetic fields 28
Emperor's Supreme Command of the
    Realm 153
emphysema 111
energy **21-43**
    blocks 23, 24, 45, 47, **48-50**, 54-5, 147, 186
    channels 28, 30, 84, 134
    environmental 33

fields 25-7, 29, 50, 132, 134
flow 24, 29, 33-4, 43, 45, 48, 54, 56, 69, 84, 153
    harmonizing 76
    physical 11
    sexual 11-12, 21, 26, 30, **32-8**, 43, 50, 57, 73, 84, 103, 108, 141
    spiritual 11-12, 21, 36, 43
    Yin and Yang 22, 23, 24, 43, 177
Energy Wave Motion Chart 85
enjoyment see joy and humour
enlightenment 15, 50, 52
erections 155, 164-5
    inability 160
eroticism 55, 62
excitation 35, 42-3, 84, 150, 160
exercise 26
eyesight and eye strain 94, 123, 177, 179, 187

fear 59, 98, 141
fetal resemblance 173
fidelity 58-9
Fire 24-5, 143, 146, 179
Five Elements Theory 21, **24-5**
    associated organs and emotions 24-5
Flat Hand Stroke 77, 78, **80**, 107, 115, 118, 143, 150
Flying on the Land **158-9**, 187
focusing 15, 36, 43, 57, 65, 67, 74
    see also visualizing
forehead 76, 174, 183, 184
Four Basic Hand Positions **77-83**
    see also Flat Hand Stroke; One Finger
    Stroke; Percussion; Pulling Stroke
Freud, Sigmund 12
frigidity 160, 187
Fuelling the Middle Burner **178**
futons 62

Gall Bladder Channel 125
    energy 178
Gate of Mortality 99, **127**
Gate of the Spine 104
genital contact 149, 159
genitals 36, 46-8, 57, 73, 99, 104, 105, 113, 116, 118, 143, 171
giver - positions and roles **73-4**
Grasping the Jaw **180**
gratification 57, 73, 102
Great Way of the Universe 13
Greeting the Five *144*, **145**
grounding the energies 123

hand positions and techniques
  see Four Basic Hand Positions
Happy Point 184
harmonizing 52, 73, 75, 161, 168
Harmonizing Fire and Water, Part I
  143, 187
Harmonizing Fire and Water, Part II
  150-1, *152*, 187
Harmonizing the Whole **168-9**, *170*
harmony 23, 30, 48, 52
headaches 76, 94, 138, 153, 174, 187
healing 26, 54, 73, 75, 88, 104, 186
  commands 76
  contact 171
  energy 21, 69, 73, 75-6, 86
  light 184
health 16, 34
heart 25, 101
  energy 111
heart centre 101, **132-3**, 142
Heart Channel 109
Heart Protector Channel 145
heat energy 76
hedonism 55-7
herbology 75, 186
hormonal release 59
hormones 51, 63
human energy field **26-7**
hypertension 187

impotence 105, 112, 187
improving low energy 161, 187
incense 62
indigestion 187
infidelity 58
inhibitions 45-6, 153
  freeing of 98, 124, 142
  guilt and shame 47, 58, 118
inner opposites **52**
insomnia 111, 187
intellect and intelligence 15, 32, 48
intercourse 35, 105
intestines 109
intuition 77, 175

Jade Pagoda 153
jaw 180
jealousy 59
Jiggling the Column **102-3**, 187
joy and humour 17, 40, 56, 111, 149, 186
Joyous Fire of the Heart 111, 115
Jung, Carl 51

Kidney Channel 125
  energy 42, 109, 113, 119, 173, 178,

179
kidneys 25, 33, 101, 109, 115-16, 141, 179
Kirlian photography 28

labia 150, 160
Leading the Fire **146**
Leading the Water **124-5**, *128*, 187
life force 11, 26, 84
limb disorders 104-5, 161, 187
liver 25, 109
Liver Channel 125
  energy 135, 178
longevity 161
lower back problems 104-5, 112, 161
lungs 25, 95, 101
lust 55, 56, 58, 158

magnetic healing energy 75-6
magnetic power 121
magnetism 160
Making an Agreement **65**, 127
male and female principle **51**
manic disorders 111
martial arts 15
massage oils 61-2, **63-4**, 138, 162
  Aphrodisia oil - recipe 63
massage sequences 77, 84-5, **94-186**
  Preparation Sequence 84, **94-9**
  Back Sequence **100-29**
  Front Sequence 70, **132-171**
  Final Sequence **172-185**
  Shortened Sequence 186
masturbation 54, 163
meditation 15, 33, **35-6**, 38, 42-3, **56-7**,
  65, 86
  Navel Breathing Meditation 36, 61, **67**
  Integrated Meditation 67
  The natural breath 67
  Posture Meditation 36, 40, 61, **66**, 70
Meeting of One Hundred Energies 99
menstruation 138, 187
mental and physical disorder 12
meridians see channels
Metal 24-5
Middle Burner **178**
migraine 177
mind-set 61
Mixing the Original and Joyous Fires
  115-16, *117*
muscle tension 101
Mysterious Passageway **174**
mystical union **35-7**

Navel Breathing Meditation 36, 61, **67**
  Integrated Meditation 67

The natural breath 67
neck pain 187
negativity 46-7, 54, 100, 103
nervous system 137, 138
nipples 151

oils see massage oils
One Finger Stroke 77, 78, **81**
oneness 15, 36, 40, 43, 59, 76, 84
Opening or Closing the Gate of Mortality
  127
Opening the Door of the Crimson Palace
  148, **149**
Opening the Doors to the Mysterious
  Passageway **174-5**, 187
Opening the Gate of the Spine **105**
Opening the Gate of Trust - for Men
  164-5
Opening the Gate of Trust - for Women
  163
optimism 173
Orbiting the Sun and Moon *176*, **177**, 187
orgasm of the valley 43
orgasms 15, 30, 42-3, 45, 84, 126, 158
  inability 153, 187
  spontaneous 166
  suppression 42
Original and Supreme Consciousness 174
Original Fire at the Gate of the Spine 112,
  174
Original Fire of Life 113
Original Fire of the Sacrum 115
Original Spirit 183
osteopathic treatment 112

palpitations 111
pancreatic energy 178
passion 48, 142
peaks and plateaus 127, 129, 145, 157-8
penis 42, 151, 164-5, 167
Percussion 77, **78**, 111, 113, 180
perineum 32, 99, 118, 126, 151, 163, 168
persona 181
pheromones 63
pituitary gland 174-5
planes of existence 30-31, 38
pleasure 45, 55-6
Posture Meditation 36, 40, 61, **66**, 70
Pounding the Door of the Mysterious
  Passageway *182*, **183**
Pounding the Doors of the Crimson
  Palace **142**
Pounding the Gate of the Spine **112-13**,
  114, 187
Pounding the Rear Door of the Crimson
  Palace *110*, **111**, 187

preparing the physical space **62**
preparing your mental space **65**
prostate gland disorders 104-5
psyche 16, 30, 51
psychic centre of consciousness 132
Pulling Stroke 77, 78, **82**
Pulling the Hips **99**
Pulling the Lower Abdomen **98**
Pulling the Temples **94**, 96
Pulling the Upper Abdomen **97**
Pulling the Upper Chest **95**
puritanism 55

receiver - positions and roles 69, **70-1**
reflected behaviour 52
reframing your sexual experience **35-6**
Reich, Wilhelm 12
relationships 45
    longstanding 58-9
    sexual 35
    with others **55-7**
    with self **46-54**
relaxation and inner peace 35, 56, 62, 65,
    84, 155, 185
religion and sexuality 46
Removing the Mask **181**
resentment and anger 180
respiratory system 116
    disorders 142, 187
Resting Positions 69, **86**
    Forehead - Final Position **184**
    Hand Between Shoulder Blades **100**
    Hands on Temples *156*, **157**
    Heart Centre **132-3**
    Holding the Pelvis **171**
    Inner Ankles **158**
    Lower Abdomen **141**
    Outer Ankle *122*, **123**
    Sacrum **104**
    Solar Plexus **137**
    Top of Thighs **121**

sacrum 32, 66, 76, 86, 102-3, 104, 112-3,
    116, 171
smell, scents, and perfumes 63, 65
sciatica 104-5
scrotum 151, 164
Sea of Blood 161
Sea of Vigour 161
Sea of Vitality 50, 138
self love 54
self massage 54
semen 42
senses 65 *see also* smell, touch
sensuousness 46, 155, 164
sex

education 45
    glands and organs 109, 175
sexual energy *see* Ching Chi
    arousal and stimulation 105, 141, 145,
    174
    drive 161
    energy levels 121
    fire 109, 139, 161
    repression 98
    stagnation 12
    trauma 104-5
sexuality 32, **44-59**
    hetero- and homosexuals 12
shoulders 73, 168
sinuses 94, 174, 178
solar plexus 57, 97, **137**
Sons of Reflected Light 13
space, mental and physical **61-7**
sperm 13, 43
spinal column and pathway 32, 36, 67,
    73-4, **101-8**, 153, 174
spirituality 11
    awareness 32, 48
    union 30
spleen 25, 109, 135
Spleen Channel 125, 160, **161**
    energy 178
sternum 132
stiff neck 153
Stirring the Water **126-7**
Stomach Channel 125, 160, **161**
    energy 178
Strengthening the Will **179**
stress 42, 94, 178
Supporting the Column Part I **108**
Supporting the Column Part II **118-19**,
    120
Supreme Commander 155

tachycardia 111
Tan T'iens **32-4**, 38, 42, 47-8, 50
    see also Divine Centres
Tao 24, 43, 52, 59, 73, 76,
    consciousness 38
    energy 73
Taoism **11-17**, 21-43, 51-2
    aims 15
    middle path 56
    beliefs 22, 26, 38, 43, 55, 173, 177
    healing wisdom 12
    medicine 25, 26, 32, 75, 103, 184
    philosophy and teachings 13, 16, 21, 25,
    30, 32, 36, 76,
    practice and techniques 15, 47
temples 157
Ten Thousand Things
    see Five Elements

tension 45, 55, 61, 147, 178
    release 35, 98, 102, 106, 108, 142, 146,
    180
testosterone 63
thymus gland 95
timing **88-9**
tongue 36
tonifiers 163, 167, 173
torso 67
touch 77, 86, 125
toxins 54
trance state 61, 65
translation of Taoist names 16
transmutation of energy 11, 12, 21, **34**,
    129
Turning the Fire - for Men **167**
Turning the Fire - for Women **166**

universe and creative energy 13, 21-6, 36,
    38
upper back region 153
urinary problems 105, 112
uterine problems 104-5

vagina 163, 166
vaginismus 105, 112, 187
vaginitis 160
vertebrae 66, 103, 107, 153
visualization 65, 97, 155, 160
    see also focusing
visualizing the energy 105-6, 139
vitality 32-4, 48, 107, 147, 173

Water 24-5, 143, 146
    energy 109
Watering the Flowers of the Kidneys *172*,
    173
Waters of Sexual Vitality 126
Wood 24-5
Wu Chi (The Absolute) 30
Wu Wei 38-40, 86

Yin and Yang 21, **22-5**, 51-2, 55
    and the eyes 177
    Channels 125
    characteristics 22-3
    dichotomy 55
    energies 22, 24, 43, 177
    blocks 23
    related illnesses 23
yoga 15